NURSING H

OFFIC
AMERICAN ASSOCIAT

ISSN 1062-8061
ISBN 978-0-8261-4362-4

2019—Volume 27

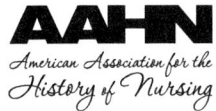

American Association for the
History of Nursing

CONTENTS

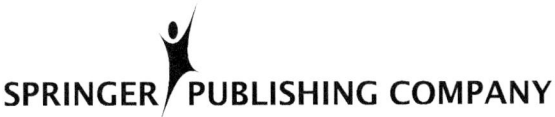

SPRINGER PUBLISHING COMPANY

NEW YORK

FESTSCHRIFT FOR SUSAN REVERBY

NOTES AND DOCUMENTS

IN MEMORIAM

MEDIA REVIEWS

REVIEW ESSAY

Book Reviews

Cover photo: "Unidentified nurse, MC 78, Mercy Douglass Hospital records." Barbara Bates Center for the Study of the History of Nursing, School of Nursing, University of Pennsylvania.

Nursing History Review is published annually for the American Association for the History of Nursing, Inc., by Springer Publishing Company, LLC, New York.

Business Office: All business correspondence, including subscriptions, renewals, advertising, and address changes, should be sent to Springer Publishing Company, LLC, 11 West 42nd Street, New York, NY 10036.

Editorial Office: Submissions and editorial correspondence should be directed to Patricia D'Antonio, Editor, *Nursing History Review*, University of Pennsylvania School of Nursing, 407 Claire M. Fagin Hall, 418 Curie Boulevard, Philadelphia, PA 19104-6096. See Guidelines for contributors on page 6 for further details.

Members of the American Association for the History of Nursing, Inc. (AAHN) receive *Nursing History Review* on payment of annual membership dues. Applications and other correspondence relating to AAHN membership should be directed to: Brian Riggs, Executive Director, American Association for the History of Nursing, Inc., P.O. Box 7, Mullica Hill, NJ 08062. Phone: 609-519-9689. E-mail: aahn@aahn.org.

Subscription Rates (per Year): For institutions: Print, $232; Online, $209; Print & Online, $336. For individuals: Print, $136; Online, $123; Print & Online, $197. Outside the United States—for institutions: Print, $258; Online, $209; Print & Online, $362. For individuals: Print, $149; Online, $123; Print & Online, $211. Payment must be made in advance by check (in U. S. dollars drawn on a U.S. bank) or international money order, payable to Springer Publishing Company, LLC, or by MasterCard, Visa, or American Express.

Indexes/abstracts of articles appear in: CINAHL® print index & database, Current Contents/ Social & Behavioral Science, Social Sciences Citation Index, Research Alert, RNdex, Index Medicus/MEDLINE, History Abstracts, America; History and Life.

Postmaster: Send address change to Springer Publishing Company, LLC, 11 West 42nd Street, New York, NY 10036.

ISSN 1062-8061

ISBN 978-0-8261-4362-4

NURSING HISTORY REVIEW GUIDELINES FOR CONTRIBUTORS

The *Nursing History Review*, the official publication of the American Association for the History of Nursing, is a peer-reviewed journal, published annually. Original research manuscripts are welcomed in broad areas related to the history of nursing, health care, health policy, and society. The *Review* defines original research as that based on primary sources, that engage with relevant sources contextualizing events and arguments in the secondary historical literature, and in ways that allow the author to make novel interpretations. The *Review* prefers manuscripts of approximately 12,000 words, inclusive of endnotes.

The *Review* regularly publishes articles that later appear as chapters in books. Our publisher, Springer Publishing, holds copyright and the author and/or publisher must formally request permission to reprint the article at http://www.springerpub.com/permission-requests. The article must predate the publication of the book.

Conflicts of Interest

Authors must inform the editors of any institutional or organizational funding that has supported research related to the manuscript. This must also be indicated in the manuscript's acknowledgements

Wellcome Trust

The publisher of the *Review* understands that research supported by the *Trust* are obligated to post final versions in a *Wellcome Trust* approved archive. Editors will continue to work with the *Trust's* requirements, *but authors must notify the editors upon submission of the manuscript.*

Preparing Your Manuscript

All authors should familiarize themselves with Springer Publishing Company Journals Policies and statements (http://www.springerpub.com/journals-policies-and-statements/)

Manuscripts must be prepared using the guidelines specified in the most recent edition of the *Chicago Manual of Style*.

Manuscripts must be double-spaced and of letter-quality print. They must also use a type size of at least 12 characters per inch or 12 points. Please leave generous margins of at least 1 inch. All pages, including text, notes, and reference pages, must be numbered consecutively. All notes must be double-spaced and placed at the end of the manuscript as endnotes rather than footnotes.

Authors are responsible for securing permissions for all materials submitted. Authors will be asked to verify that they have secured written permission for publication of any interview or oral history data. If more than 500 words of text are quoted from a book, or more than 250 words from an article, or if a table or figure has been previously published, the manuscript must be accompanied by written permission from the copyright owner. Quoting from an unpublished thesis can be particularly challenging. If an author quotes more than five lines from such an unpublished thesis, he or she needs to provide a letter granting permission from either the author or the sponsoring institution.

Initial submissions of manuscripts must use *Editorial Manager* http://www.editorialmanager.com/NHR/default.aspx . This system will ask for the relevant information about titles, authors, abstracts, key words, and manuscript. If applicable, acknowledgements can be included on your title page. *Editorial Manager* will also ask for a copyright agreement, with the printed notice that if a manuscript is rejected, copyright returns to the author

Final versions of manuscripts accepted for publication will also be uploaded through *Editorial Manager.* Photographs or other figures accompanying the final manuscript must be attached in *Editorial Manager* as TIF files with resolutions of at least 600 dpi.

Author's Biographical Information

Manuscripts

The final version of an accepted manuscript should include a <u>brief </u>author biographical sketch at the end of the text of the manuscript with the author's name capitalized

For example: PATRICIA D'ANTONIO is the Killebrew-Censits Term Professor, Chair of the Department of Family and Community Health, and Director of the

Barbara Barbara Bates Center for the Study of the History of Nursing at the University of Pennsylvania School of Nursing. She is the author of *American Nursing: A History of Knowledge, Authority and the Meaning of Work* (Baltimore: The Johns Hopkins University Press, 2010) and *Nursing with a Mission: Public Health in New York City* (New Brunswick: The Rutgers University Press, 2017)

You may include an e-mail address here if you so choose

Book and Media Reviews

Book and media reviews will currently stay outside *Editorial Manager* as we adjust to the system. Your editors will give you instructions about how to format the introduction of your reviews. You should only give your name, credentials, and academic or organizational affiliation at the end.

Most correspondence about manuscripts will remain in *Editorial Manager*. Other correspondence can be sent to: Patricia D'Antonio, PhD, RN, FAAN, Editor, *Nursing History Review*, University of Pennsylvania School of Nursing, 407 Claire M. Fagin Hall, 418 Curie Boulevard, Philadelphia, PA 19104-6096. Phone: 215/746.4188. Fax: 215/573-2168. E-mail: *dantonio@nursing.upenn.edu* or *nhr@nursing.upenn.edu* . All correspondence regarding book or media reviews should be sent to your relevant editor.

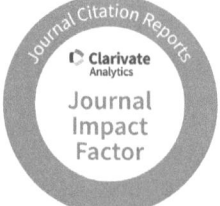

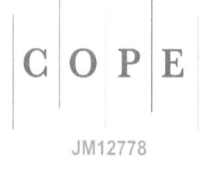

JM12778

EDITOR'S NOTE

Publish or Perish—and Your Peril

We have all heard about the dangerousness of predatory publishers: those that promise immediate, peer-reviewed publication of any manuscript on any subject just for the payment of a "small" (and, in reality, not so small) fee. The pressure in global academia, especially the new pressure to publish in English language journals, has given rise to commercial publishers literally inventing journals to meet this need. Almost every day we are all inundated with notices of new journals (many with names that seem eerily familiar) that are looking to publish or reprint our scholarship. Do we really have the energy to concentrate on differentiating *Research on Health and Nursing* from *Research on Nursing and Health*, a prestigious peer reviewed journal edited by Eileen Lake? The name predatory accurately reflects the way these for-profit publishers prey on the pressures academics experience on an almost daily basis.

For the last several years, editors of nursing journals have been steadfastly campaigning to ensure that scholars in the discipline and, as importantly, their students do not fall prey to the sophisticated snares of predatory publishers. We have written editorials, spoken at conferences, and counselled new authors. I thought we were making headway.

We are not. *Bealls List*, a once reliable guide to predatory journals and their publishers, has been taken off the Internet. What I once saw as a problem for our international colleagues has come to the shores of the United States. At the last meeting of the International Academy of Nurse Editors, participants spoke of reference lists that included journals of which they—as specialists—have never heard and that could not be verified. I have reviewed promotion dossiers that included articles from unrecognized journals which, upon investigation, promise quick publication upon payment. And, as editor of the *Nursing History Review*, I have responded to irritated authors demanding to know why a submission has not been accepted for publication within 72 hours.

These predatory journals promote themselves as conventional publication vehicles. And I use the word "conventional" deliberately. I watch with

Nursing History Review 27 (2019): 12–14. A Publication of the American Association for the History of Nursing. Copyright © 2019 Springer Publishing Company.
http://dx.doi.org/10.1891/1062-8061.27.12

interest—and have even begun to participate in—the emergence of social media sites as new places to disseminate and debate new scholarship. I believe we will see more and more of these different kinds of ways to build scholarship. I call attention only to journals which masquerade as what we recognize as the gold standard of scholarly dissemination.

But there has been one important change: there has been enough attention to this issue in the nursing literature—through editorials and research surveys about the extent to which articles in these publications have permeated the discipline's discourse—that scholars can no longer pretend a certain innocence or ignorance about where they choose to publish. The responsibility—and the attendant reputational impact—now lies solely with us.

I am somewhat reluctant to discuss a second concern in an editorial in which I rail about the perils of predatory publications. So let me be clear: I am now switching topics to what I see as a problematic but not illegitimate publishing practice. Many of our universities are now encouraging the publication of our scholarship on institutional sites often called *Creative Commons*. Publishers generally allow this after they have accepted a manuscript for publication, and most make processes for uncorrected page proofs to be posted on this public site prior to official publication (please do check with individual publishers about relevant policies and procedures). My concerns lie with our students. In many places, the default setting upon the deposit of a dissertation is to make the content immediately available. This works well to support the vibrancy of an institution's educational mission. The issue lies in the current debate among editors as to whether or not this constitutes prior publication: if it does, then the relevant manuscript chapter from a dissertation is automatically precluded from publication in a conventional journal. This issue is as yet unsettled.

But if you will allow me a few more sentences on my editorial soapbox, I will argue that we need to make sure we protect ourselves and our students. All dissertations need to be embargoed until publication plans are finalized. This is particularly urgent for historical dissertations that may later appear as a book. I have experienced publishers who have refused to consider book length manuscripts because the material is essentially available for free download on Creative Commons sites.

It is a brave new world out there. It is exciting as new forms of scholarly dissemination appear. But it is also a place of peril if we do not approach dissemination with caution. A final word: if something appears too good to be true, it probably is.

What has really been too good to be true was Brigid Lusk's tenure as one of the *Review*'s book review editor. Brigid came to the *Review* in her retirement and, after many years of strong service, has decided that retirement really should mean less rather than more commitments. On behalf of the entire editorial team and the readership of the *Review*, I sincerely thank her for her service. And, knowing Brigid, we can look forward to hearing about her next great adventure when we meet in San Diego.

Patricia D'Antonio, PhD, RN, FAAN
Barbara Bates Center for the Study of the History of Nursing
University of Pennsylvania School of Nursing
407 Claire Fagin Hall
418 Curie Boulevard
Philadelphia, PA 19104-4217

INAUGURAL LORRAINE ALBRECHT LECTURE
UNIVERSITY OF VIRGINIA ELEANOR CROWDER BJORING CENTER FOR HISTORICAL NURSING INQUIRY

Hidden and Forgotten: Being Black in the American Red Cross Town and Country Nursing Service, 1912–1948

SANDRA B. LEWENSON
Pace University

Early 20th-century morbidity and mortality rates show that African Americans in rural communities fared far worse than their white counterparts.[1] While all populations living in rural settings shared a lack of access to health care due to difficult travel over poor roads, an insufficient number of health care providers willing to deal with working in isolated settings, and too often the effects of poverty, health care disparities were further compounded by race. To improve rural health care in the United States—especially for white rural populations—the American Red Cross (ARC) between 1912 and 1948 experimented with the notion of using its vast quasi national organization to support local communities to develop public health nursing structures. The ARC established the Town and Country Nursing Service to accomplish this goal.[2] This unique experiment in peacetime health care advocacy, from its inception, found it difficult to attract white-educated nurses with the required rural public health training to leave the cities for rural communities. It was

Nursing History Review 27 (2019): 15–28. A Publication of the American Association for the History of Nursing. Copyright © 2019 Springer Publishing Company.
http://dx.doi.org/10.1891/1062-8061.27.15

near impossible to find black nurses who fit the educational requirements of the ARC. The racist attitudes of schools of nursing in the north and south—although varied due to custom or law[3]—limited the number of black nurses who could fulfill the requirement of the ARC's experiment in establishing rural nursing services. Even more challenging for black nurses' acceptance into the service was the ARC's practice of maintaining the status quo of segregation within communities and within the military.

While little is known about the ARC rural nursing experience in general, even less is known of the black nurses who sought to serve in the rural communities. These women remained hidden and forgotten, often omitted from historical accounts. My article focuses on searching out the hidden and forgotten African American nurses who served in the ARC rural nursing service and exploring the barriers they faced in their efforts to serve. As I began to investigate this topic, I found that few records remain of these women and as a result it was difficult to determine how many black rural public health nurses actually served—especially in the early years of the organization, and who they were. One person, however, stands in the records whom I will focus on in this article. The first known African American public health nurse accepted into the Town and Country Nursing Service was Frances Elliot Davis. Davis entered the Town and Country in 1917 and received the ARC badge number 1-A in 1918. She appeared first on a separate list of nurses where "A" designated race. The ARC established this list in 1918 and maintained it throughout both World Wars ending its practice in 1949.[4]

In this article, I argue that black nurses, in particular, faced discriminatory practices rooted in societal norms, as a result of their gender, their race, and their professional role. I examine the barriers black nurses faced in entering the Red Cross including admission policies and segregation practices. It is well documented that racial bias, segregation, and discrimination limited the black nurses' experience in all areas of nursing and health care during the early part of the 20th century.[5] This article, however, expands on this work by using the ARC Town and Country Nursing Service and its limited acceptance of African American nurses as a case study. It reflects upon the one black nurse known to be accepted into the Town and Country in 1917, 5 years after the start of the organization. In addition, as a result of the US entry into World War I in that same year, the acceptance of black nurses into the ARC becomes part of the broader story because of the gatekeeper role the ARC played in supplying nurses into the Army Nurses Corps, the Navy Nurse Corps, and the US Public Health Service. While this article focuses mostly on Frances Elliot Davis and the Town and Country, it cannot help but touch upon the practice of separating the nursing recruits by color—using a separate list to identify black nursing recruits beginning in 1918—in order to maintain the status quo of segregation in public health and active service.

Background of the Town and Country Nursing Service

The Town and Country Nursing Service began in 1912. It had been conceived a few years earlier by Lillian D. Wald, the noted public health nursing leader and founder of the Henry Street Settlement on the Lower East Side of New York City. Her vision to improve the health of all Americans extended to those populations living in rural communities as well as in urban centers. She found financial backers to join her in convincing the ARC to expand its mission to address the health care needs of the nation in times of peace, as well as during manmade and natural disasters. The ARC Rural Nursing Service (as it was called that first year) began in 1912.[6] By the following year, to reflect the inclusion of small towns along with rural communities, its name changed to the Town and Country Nursing Service. Over the next 36 years of its existence, the organization and its name continued to evolve, in order to address the needs of a nation during war, peace, economic hard times, and epidemics. The record showed that during its lifetime, over "3,109 public health nursing services in about 1,800 counties under the sponsorship of some 2,100 chapters" was provided.[7]

ARC rural nurses served in communities throughout the Unites States, which required the ability to work in isolated areas, where roads were scarce, and local customs strong. These nurses needed good communication skills in order to collaborate with interested stakeholders often including local school boards, rural physicians, businesses, women's clubs, and church groups. They needed skills to educate the community about sanitation, public health promotion, water safety and the like. This required additional education that included the skill sets these nurses would need working in these rural areas and small towns, where the resources found in urban settings were limited and unavailable. ARC rural public health nurses would be required to include additional education, not only at the postgraduate level following their 3-year diploma program, but also at least 2 years of high school prior to attending nurses' training. Fannie Clement, first director of the Town and Country Nursing Service wrote in the *American Journal of Nursing* that "all future candidates will be expected to have a minimum of 2 years of high school … the responsibilities developing upon the isolated workers in the small communities indicate the need of the best educated women."[8] Although the requirement of a high school diploma by the end of 1916 was voted on by the Town and Country, this criterion was waived due to the impending involvement in World War I and the nurse shortage that it caused making it even more difficult to attract more nurses to the ARC rural nursing service.[9]

Admission Requirements

The ARC required a "minimum age of 25, a doctor's certificate with renewal every 2 years, and a certificate of registration in states where registration was required and in other states graduate from a recognized school of nursing with a course of not less than 2 years."[10] With the exception of age, all Town and Country nurses needed to meet these basic ARC requirements. In addition to these, nurses had to show they had successfully completed a 4-month (at the minimum) course in public health nursing. This additional requirement often stood in the way of attracting nurses into this service due to the additional expense and the time it required.[11] To attract nurses, the Town and Country established scholarships to meet the postgraduate requirement. These scholarships offered economic support and incentive for those nurses willing to work in rural communities that lacked roads, access to health services, or comforts of city living.

During the winter of 1913–1914, Teachers College in New York City's Columbia University offered one of the early postgraduate 4-month courses that fulfilled the educational requirement of the Town and Country.[12] The curriculum evolved to include a practicum in rural health with the District Nursing Association of Westchester County and urban health at the Henry Street Settlement in New York City. Courses covered a wide array of relevant topics touching on rural health, preventive medicine, public health nursing, and rural and urban sanitation.[13] These educational programs prepared Town and Country nurses with a wide array of skills needed in order to provide care for the sick, as well as the health promotion and disease prevention desperately needed in rural settings. The courses prepared these nurses to hone their communication skills necessary to work with other professionals and the public when establishing the public health nursing services in a particular community.

Few programs offered postgraduate coursework in public health, and even fewer prior to 1917 were offered by schools in the south. Yet even with scholarships and programs available, black nurses faced barriers to attending these programs. The Canadian nurse educator, Ethel Johns authored a 1925 unpublished report for the Rockefeller Foundation titled, "A Study of the Present Status of the Negro Woman in Nursing." In this report, she described the existence of serious racial bias in most schools of nursing that she felt could not be ignored. Even in some postgraduate programs in northern universities that typically admitted black students, their welcome she said was, "far from enthusiastic."[14]

This lack of enthusiasm to admit black nurses in most of the public health programs could be found in the responses to letters that Katharine W. Holmes, assistant director of the newly named ARC rural nursing service in the Bureau of Public Health Nursing, received. Holmes had written to postgraduate programs in public health about their admission policies regarding race. Anne H. Strong at Boston's Simmons College responded that it makes "no restriction as to race or color."[15] However, she relayed an experience with a black student, who although was fully qualified to be admitted, once admitted was "not successful," even though in the end she received her certification. Based on her experience, Strong wrote that she "would never advise colored students to come here for training," but, if they did, she would do her best to assist them in the program. One of the barriers highlighted by Strong was that the field work required extra effort, as well as the special living arrangements for black students. Also, Strong explained, that there was little demand to hire "colored nurses, and the one whom I have just mentioned finally went back to private duty."[16] After receiving several similar responses in other letters, Holmes candidly wrote it, "makes me wish courses in public health nursing were a little more flexible in regards to their qualifications for admission in so far as the color of the nurse is concerned."[17]

Three years earlier in 1917, Frances Elliot (Davis) received one of the early educational scholarships from the Red Cross to attend the course at Teachers College in preparation for her acceptance into the Town and Country. Teachers College was one of the few schools to admit black nurses into their program. Her early training school experience at Freedman's School of Nursing in Washington, DC (where she graduated in 1912 or 1913 depending on the source)[18] along with the passage of state registration, qualified her to apply and be accepted into the ARC on July 30, 1917.[19] Following the completion of her postgraduate course at Teachers College, she spent her subsequent time at the Henry Street Settlement while waiting for an assignment where a black nurse would be accepted. Davis was finally sent to Jackson, Tennessee. Davis did not receive the ARC badge 1-A for another year, while the ARC tried to figure out the placement of black nurses.

The discrepancy in the year long wait for the Red Cross Badge may have to do with the general status of nurses in the Town and Country, as well as race. As public health nursing activist Lavinia Dock explained, "not all Town and Country nurses were necessarily 'enrolled'"[20] in the active Red Cross service. Town and Country nurses wore a Red Cross pendant, rather than the Red Cross badge when admitted. However, when the United States entered the World War I in April 1917, many of the Town and Country nurses wanted to volunteer in the war effort. But fearful of losing public health nurses to the general population, Red Cross *Bulletin* reported that same month, that Town and Country nurses would not be called into war service unless they were drastically needed.[21] Their work in rural public health was considered valuable to the nation and therefore, to the Red Cross. However, Frances Elliot Davis, as far as the records show, was the only identifiable black nurse who was admitted into the Town and Country. While records are unclear here, she had seemingly requested a move into active service but had to wait until the ARC could figure out where to place her for service.

Gatekeepers

The ARC served as gatekeeper for nurses who wanted to enter the Army Nurse Corps, as well as the Navy Nurse Corps and the US Public Health Service. The Army Nurse Corps maintained the Army's practice of segregation, so that when black nurses were finally admitted into the Army Nurse Corps in July 1918 they were enrolled but only in the reserve. They were not expected to be engaged in active duty as a result of the lack of segregated quarters available to black nurses.[22] Adah Thoms, President of the National Association of Colored Graduate Nurses, had written to ARC nursing director Jane Delano, advocating the inclusion of black nurses into the Army Nurse Corps. Delano, in turn, wrote to Dora E. Thompson, Superintendent of the Army Nurse Corps as to what the "probability" was for the Surgeon General to assign black nurses to active service.[23] Thompson wrote back immediately:

> In reply to your letter of December 18, 1917 relative to colored nurses, so far as I know there is no immediate prospect of calling upon them for duty. I think it might be advisable to enroll them, as should the need arise later they would be available for service, but they should be enrolled with the understanding that their assignment is an uncertain proposition.[24]

The question of admission of blacks into the Red Cross continued—although the policy established earlier in 1911 prohibiting blacks from entering due to segregation in the armed forces was later lifted in 1917 when the need for black nurses superseded racial bias.[25] On June 10, 1918, Delano informed the Division Directors about the authorization of "colored nurses." She already had a list of possible nurses who would be eligible for enrollment, and their names would be sent to the local committees for their endorsement based on the usual requirements. Anyone who applied directly to the local committees should be "listed as colored, so that in the enrollment here [*sic*] may be no possibility of assigning them to duty without reference to their color…We shall issue a new series of badges marked 1-A, 2-A, 3-A, etc., and file their applications in a separate file as colored nurses."[26] One month later, Delano again explained the change in practice writing that now the Red Cross was:

> …enrolling colored nurses for service, and already have colored nurses in the Town and Country Nursing Service, and in the Sanitary Zones, so that as far as the Department of Nursing is concerned, we shall be entirely willing to make arrangements for the assignment to duty of a colored nurse if it meets with the approval of the Public Health Officials.[27]

On July 2, 1918, a year after Frances Elliot Davis had joined the ARC Town and Country, she received her badge 1-A—the first nurse to be included on an enrollment list where the "A" referred to her race. Davis thus became known as the first African American nurse to receive such a designation, and although in later years, this was questioned, the designation has remained.

After receiving her ARC badge with 1-A stamped on the back, Frances Elliot Davis, was assigned to Chattanooga, Tennessee (and then to Jackson, Tennessee) to provide public health services in the cantonment zone surrounding the army bases. Public health nurses, like Davis, were assigned to protect the health of civilian populations.[28] Davis's placement in the newspaper listed her as part of the US Public Health Service, Unit number 16. Following the armistice in November 1918, she left active duty, although remained in the Red Cross reserve (personal email communication with Jean Shulman). Her work brought her to Detroit, Michigan at Dunbar hospital, where Davis started one of the first schools of nursing for black women in the state of Michigan. Davis later returned to public health work working for the Detroit Visiting Nurse Service and the Detroit Department of Public Health and she lived in Mount Clemens, Michigan.[29] The only biography about Davis by Jean Maddern Pitrone indicated that in 1929 she returned to Teachers College for a baccalaureate degree in nursing but she was unable to complete her degree due to illness.[30]

Persistent racism followed Frances Elliott Davis even after she had died in May 2, 1965. Although she was to receive an award by the Red Cross for her service later that year, some of the office records questioned whether or not she was the first black nurse to serve. Her biographer, Pitrone, was informed by the Red Cross headquarters in the 1960s that another nurse, Georgia Hall from Topeka, Kansas had been admitted as the first black nurse into the ARC and was given badge number 19041. The ARC Enrollment Records (n.d.) that were kept at the ARC indicated that Georgia Hall was issued the badge number 19041 in error but "…it was decided not to recall the badge."[31] In 1968 Red Cross official, Ramon Eaton, settled the issue by writing that Davis was the first black nurse in the ARC. He refuted the notion that black nurses entered the ARC Town and Country prior to her admission, most emphatically explaining "…that any Negro nurses who applied for enrollment as a Negro would have been turned down prior to the date of Mrs. Davis' enrollment."[32]

Conclusion

The barriers that black nurses faced in entering the Town and Country and later practices where only six black nurses were reportedly admitted in the renamed Bureau of Public Health Nursing, along with the exclusion of blacks from active service during the war, spurred these nurses to look elsewhere to provide the much-needed public health services to their communities.[33] The Circle for Negro War Relief, for example, was formed in 1917 for the purpose of caring for black soldiers and their families and was reorganized in 1919 to address public health issues.[34] Attempts were made to establish links with the Blue Circle Public Health nurses to the ARC, but this did not come to fruition. In 1920, the Director of the Bureau of Red Cross, Elizabeth Fox, wrote to Arthur B. Spingarn, representing the Blue Circle saying that,

> …[we] appreciate the fact that situations may arise in which racial prejudice is the dominating factor. We believe that such situations are growing less and that the white members of a community are becoming more and more conscious of the fact that it is poor economy to dis-regard the needs and welfare of the colored population, to say nothing of its in-humanity.[35]

Black nurses were excluded due to laws codifying segregation in the south and unrelenting racist attitudes, both conscious and unconscious, in the north and south that permeated the policies of the ARC. These nurses were further challenged by commonly held beliefs that black nurses received an inferior education, and therefore were less prepared to serve. Their ability to serve was also hampered by states that barred or discouraged African American nurses from taking the state board registration exams that made them ineligible to enter the ARC; and the assumed lack of having supervisory ability also contributed to the limitation and exclusion of these nurses.[36] Historian Darlene Clark Hine wrote that "the process of professionalization of black nursing was littered with obstacles."[37] I believe that the designation of black nurses by race on their badge was just one of those obstacles these nurses endured. That practice ended in 1949, as did the Red Cross's rural public health nursing service. However, the list may allow us to search out the many hidden and forgotten nurses who served in the ARC, public health experience.

The uncovering of Frances Elliot Davis, one of the many "hidden figures" in nursing is significant on many levels. First, it acknowledges who these women were and the context in which they lived and worked. Second, by searching out these nurses, it allows for historical reflection and analysis. Few African American nurses were identified as ARC rural nurses. This may be due to the fact that few records were kept in general of these nurses, and even fewer records were kept for black nurses. Those nurses that were deemed important to the ARC in some way found their records sent to Ancestry.com. Perhaps even more significant for us today is that to study the lives of people, like Frances Elliot Davis, we can uncover the bias, both conscious and unconscious[38] that permeates the educational and practice settings in which we work. The American Association of Colleges of Nurses as well as the American Academy of Nursing have published an inclusivity and diversity position paper calling for nurses to treat all people equally. These organizations have sought to address the known racial bias and tensions black nurses have experienced in our history overtime. The racism experienced by nurses like Frances Elliot Davis and the negative effect on health care for the black community resonate with us today.[39]

Yet, it also shows the strength of many of these women, who faced extraordinary challenges, and perhaps, I believe, resonates with Adah Thoms' message that regardless of how the world viewed them, they needed to make the world better. In her 1917 address to the National Medical Association, Thoms said "I am filled with pride to know that despite the handicaps that beset us on every side, we are moving steadily forward and when, as our president said in his wonderful masterpiece, 'that the world must be made safe for democracy,' whether he meant to include us or not makes no difference, we are included, and there is no power outside of ourselves that can keep us from sharing the liberty and freedom for which democracy stands."[40]

Acknowledgments

This research was completed in part from the funding received from the Pace University Scholarly Research Award and the Pace University Keenan Award for Travel. I also want to thank historians Julie Fairman, Barbra Mann Wall, Annemarie McAllister, and Patricia D'Antonio for their review of previous drafts of this manuscript.

Notes

1. Wileur, Creesy L. "Mortality Statistics, (1912). Thirteenth Annual Report." Vital Statistics. Department of Commerce, USA, (1913). https://www.cdc.gov/nchs/data/vsushistorical/mortstatsh_1912.pdf; Noonan, Allan S., Hector Eduardo Velasco-Mondragon, & Fernando A. Wagner. "Improving the Health of African Americans in the USA: An Overdue Opportunity for Social Justice." *Public Health Reviews 37,* no. 12 (2016): 1–20. https://doi.org/10.1186/s40985-016-0025-4.

2. The ARC rural nursing service changed its name throughout its existence to reflect changes in its scope of practice: Rural Nursing Service (1912–1913); Town and Country Nursing Service (1913–1918); Bureau of Public Health Nursing (1918–1932); Public Health Nursing and Home Hygiene and Care of the Sick (1932–1948). For a more complete discussion of the ARC evolving names, see "Town and Country Nursing: Community Participation and Nurse Recruitment." In *Nursing Rural America: Perspectives from the Early 20th Century,* 1–19. New York, NY: Springer (2015).

3. Carnegie, M. Elizabeth. *The Path We Tread: Blacks in Nursing, 1854–1994.* 3rd ed. Burlington, MA: Jones & Bartlett, (2000); Staupers, Mabel Keaton. *No Time for Prejudice: A Story of the Integration of Negros in Nursing in the United States.* New York: The Macmillan Company (1961).

4. American Red Cross. "American Red Cross Enrollment Numbers of African American Nurses, 1918–1949." unpublished, no date. (Shared with author by the ARC volunteer Jean Shulman who obtained this material at the American Red Cross Archives, National Headquarters: Washington, DC. These archives are no longer open to the public. Most of the ARC archives are in the National Archives II in College Park, MD.) (This author has developed a spreadsheet listing each of these women listed on the enrollment list.)

5. Hine, Darlene Clark. *Black Women in White: Racial Conflict and Cooperation in the Nursing Profession 1890–1950.* Bloomington, IN: Indiana University Press (1989); Threat, Charissa J. *Nursing Civil Rights: Gender and Race in the Army Nurse Corps.* Urbana, Chicago, and Springfield, IL: University of Illinois Press, (2015); Thoms, Adah B. *Pathfinders: A History of the Progress of Colored Graduate Nurses* (1929); Pitt-Mosley, Marie Oleatha. *A History of Black Leaders in Nursing: The Influence of Four Black Community Health Nurses on the Establishment, Growth, and Practice of Public Health Nurses in New York City, 1900–1930* (Ed. D. diss., Teachers College, Columbia University) (1992). http://pocketknowledge.tc.columbia.edu/home.php/viewfile/8534.

6. Dock, Lavinia, Sarah Elizabeth Pickett, Clara, D. Noyes, Fannie, F., Clement, Elizabeth G., Fox, & Anna R Van Meter. *History of American Red Cross Nursing*. New York: The Macmillan Company, (1922); Lewenson, Sandra B. "Town and Country Nursing: Community Participation and Nurse Recruitment." In *Nursing Rural America: Perspectives from the Early 20th Century*, edited by John C. Kirchgessner & Arlene W. Keeling, 1–19. New York, NY: Springer (2015); Lewenson, Sandra B. "Historical Exemplars in Nursing." In *Practicing Primary Health Care: Caring for Populations*, 1–19. Burlington, MA: Jones and Bartlett Learning, (2017).

7. Kernodle, Portia B. *The Red Cross Nurse in Action, 1882–1948*. New York: Harper & Brothers Publishers (1949), p. 469.

8. Clement, Fannie F. "The Red Cross: The American Red Cross Town and Country." *The American Journal of Nursing 15*, no. 7 (1915): 580–84, p. 583.

9. For a full discussion of the educational requirements, see Dock, Lavinia, Sarah Elizabeth Pickett, Clara D. Noyes, Fannie F. Clement, Elizabeth G. Fox, and Anna R Van Meter. *History of American Red Cross Nursing*. New York: The Macmillan Company (1922), p. 1236.

10. Minutes of the Second meeting of the Committee on Rural Nursing, December 10, 1912, p. 1, Rockefeller Sanitary Commission Microfilm, Reel 1, Folder 8 American Red Cross Town & Country Nursing Service 1912–1914. Rockefeller Archive Collection, Pocantico, NY.

11. "Minutes of the Second Meeting of the Committee on Rural Nursing," December 10, 1912, p. 1, Rockefeller Sanitary Commission Microfilm, Reel 1, Folder 8 American Red Cross Town & Country Nursing Service 1912–1914, Rockefeller Archive Center, Pocantico, NY.

12. For a description of the program at Teachers College, Columbia University in conjunction with the Henry Street Settlement and the District Nursing Service of Northern Westchester (a rural community north of New York City), see "Post Graduate Courses for Red Cross Town and Country Nursing Service Candidates (4 months course), 1914–1915," Pocket Knowledge, Department of Nursing and Health, American Red Cross Town & Country Nursing Service, Published 1899–1961, uploaded 6/15/2009 by Pocket Masters, Archives of the Department of Nursing Education, 0397.pdf file, page 2. Other 4- and 8-month programs that included rural public health courses were started at the Instructive District Nursing Association in Boston; the Visiting Nurse Association in Chicago, IL, and the Richmond Instructive Vising Nurse Association in Richmond, VA.

13. Dock, Lavinia, Sarah Elizabeth Pickett, Clara D. Noyes, Fannie F. Clement, Elizabeth G. Fox, & Anna R Van Meter. *History of American Red Cross Nursing*. New York: The Macmillan Company (1922), p. 1250.

14. Johns, Ethel. (1925). A study of the present status of the Negro woman in nursing. Rockefeller Foundation, Record Group 1.1, series 200, Box 122, Folder 1507, pp. 1–43, (quote found on p. 7). Exhibits A-P (Appendixes I and II). Rockefeller Archive Center, Pocantico, NY.

15. Letter from Anne H. Strong, School for Public Health Nursing, Simmons College and the Instructive District Nursing Association, to Katherine Holmes, Assistant Director, Red Cross Bureau of Public Health Nursing, September 20, 1920. Shared with author by the ARC volunteer Jean Shulman who obtained this material at the American Red Cross Archives, National Headquarters: Washington, DC. These archives are no longer

open to the public. Most of the ARC archives are in the National Archives and Record Administration II in College Park, MD.

16. Ibid.

17. Letter from Katherine Holmes, Assistant Director, Red Cross Bureau of Public Health Nursing to Miss Virginia Robinson, Pennsylvania School for Social Service, September 21, 1920. Shared with author by the ARC volunteer Jean Shulman who obtained this material at the American Red Cross Archives, National Headquarters: Washington, DC. These archives are no longer open to the public. Most of the ARC archives are in the National Archives II in College Park, MD.

18. It is unclear to this researcher which graduating class Davis was part of. According to Thoms (1929), the Freedman's school where Davis attended was 2 years in length and Davis entered in (1910). This would mean she would have graduated in (1912) (Coles, 1969); But the date in Pitrone's book is (1913), and in the (1960s) correspondence with the Red Cross … (1913) (Red Cross Records).

19. Coles, Anna B. "The Howard University School of Nursing in Historical Perspective." *Journal of the National Medical Association 61*, no. 2 (March 1969): 105–18. https://www.ncbi.nlm.nih.gov/pmc/articles/PMC2611690/pdf/jnma00516-0005.pdf; Thoms, Adah B. *Pathfinders: A History of the Progress of Colored Graduate Nurses*, (1929); Carnegie, M. Elizabeth. *The Path We Tread: Blacks in Nursing, 1854–1994*. 3rd ed. Burlington, MA: Jones & Bartlett (2000).

20. Dock, Lavinia, Sarah Elizabeth Pickett, Clara D. Noyes, Fannie F. Clement, Elizabeth G. Fox, and Anna R Van Meter. *History of American Red Cross Nursing*. New York: The Macmillan Company (1922), p. 1271.

21. Ibid.

22. Sarnecky, Mary T. *A History of the U.S. Army Nurse Corps*. Studies in Health, Illness, and Caregiving. Philadelphia, PA: University of Pennsylvania Press, 1999; Threat, Charissa J. *Nursing Civil Rights: Gender and Race in the Army Nurse Corps*. Urbana, Chicago, and Springfield, IL: University of Illinois Press (2015).

23. Dock, Lavinia, Sarah Elizabeth Pickett, Clara D. Noyes, Fannie F. Clement, Elizabeth G. Fox, & Anna R Van Meter. *History of American Red Cross Nursing*. New York: The Macmillan Company (1922), p. 406.

24. "Letter to Jane A. Delano, Director, Department of Nursing, ARC from Dora E. Thompson, Superintendent, Army Nurse Corps," December 19, 1917. National Archives II, American Red Cross, 300.1 Negro Nurses-Enrollment, College Park, MD.

25. Dock, Lavinia, Sarah Elizabeth Pickett, Clara D. Noyes, Fannie F. Clement, Elizabeth G. Fox, & Anna R Van Meter. *History of American Red Cross Nursing*. New York: The Macmillan Company (1922).

26. "Letter to the Division Directors from Jane A. Delano, Director, Department of Nursing, American Red Cross," June 10, 1918. 300.1. National Archives II, American Red Cross, 300.1 Negro Nurses – Enrollment, College Park, MD.

27. "Letter from Jane A. Delano, Director, Department of Nursing to Mr. Hamlen," August 20, 1918. The American Red Cross Archives (shared with author by the ARC volunteer Jean Shulman who obtained this material at the American Red Cross Archives, National Headquarters: Washington, DC. These archives are no longer open to the public. Most of the ARC archives are in the National Archives II in College Park, MD).

28. Kalisch, Phillip A., & Beatrice J. Kalisch. *Nurturer of Nurses: A History of the Division of Nursing of the U.S. Public Health Service and Its Antecedents*. Vol. Summary of Review of the Study. 5 vols. (1977), p. 2. Barbara Bates Center for the Study of the History of Nursing. University of Pennsylvania, Philadelphia, PA (materials shared with this author by Cindy Connolly, Assistant Director of the Barbara Bates Center for the Study of the History of Nursing).

29. Coles, Anna B. "The Howard University School of Nursing in Historical Perspective." *Journal of the National Medical Association 61*, no. 2 (March 1969): 105–18. https://www.ncbi.nlm.nih.gov/pmc/articles/PMC2611690/pdf/jnma00516-0005.pdf.

30. Pitrone, Jean Maddern. *Trailblazer: Negro Nurse in the American Red Cross*. New York: Harcourt, Brace & World, Inc. (1969).

31. American Red Cross. "American Red Cross Enrollment Numbers of African American Nurses, 1918–1949." unpublished, no date.

32. "Letter from Ramone Eaton to Mr. James B. Foley, Re: Mrs. Frances Reid [*sic*] Elliott Davis, R.N. '1A,'" December 11, 1968. National Archives and Record Administration (NARA), U.S. American Red Cross Nursing Files, 1915–1969. Ancestor. Com. https://search.ancestry.com/search/db.aspx?dbid=2365.

33. Hine, Darlene Clark. *Black Women in White: Racial Conflict and Cooperation in the Nursing Profession 1890–1950*. Bloomington, IN: Indiana University Press (1989), p. 106.

34. "Circle for Negro Relief-Attached to Letter by Assistant Director of the Red Cross Bureau of Public Health Nursing, to Emily W. Dinwiddle, National Headquarters and Katharine W. Holmes, Assistant Director, Bureau of Public Health Nursing," October 8, 1920. Box 45, 041.1 Circle for Negro War Relief. National Archives II, American Red Cross, RG 200, Group 2 1917–1934, College Park, MD.; also see Lewenson, Sandra Beth. *Taking Charge: Nursing Suffrage, and Feminism in America, 1873–1920*. Development of American Feminism. New York: Garland Publishing (1993).

35. "Letter to Arthur B. Spingarn, The Circle for Negro Relief from Elizabeth Fox, Director, Red Cross Bureau of Public Health Nursing." Letter, July 22, 1920 (p. 2). National Archives II, American Red Cross, RG 200, Group 2 1917–1934, Box 45, Group 2. College Park, MD (Arthur B. Spingarn was a lawyer and official in the NAACP).

36. Dock, Lavinia, Sarah Elizabeth Pickett, Clara D. Noyes, Fannie F. Clement, Elizabeth G. Fox, & Anna R Van Meter. *History of American Red Cross Nursing*. New York: The Macmillan Company (1922); Hine, Darlene Clark. *Black Women in White: Racial Conflict and Cooperation in the Nursing Profession 1890–1950*. Bloomington, IN: Indiana University Press, (1989); Johns, Ethel. (1925). A study of the present status of the Negro woman in nursing. Rockefeller Foundation, Record Group 1.1, series 200, Box 122, Folder 1507, pp. 1–43. Exhibits A-P (Appendixes I and II). Rockefeller Archive Center, Pocantico, NY.

37. Hine, Darlene Clark. *Black Women in White: Racial Conflict and Cooperation in the Nursing Profession 1890–1950*. Bloomington, IN: Indiana University Press (1989), p. 97.

38. AACN. "American Association of the Colleges of Nursing (AACN) Position Statement on Diversity, Inclusion, & Equity in Academic Nursing." *Journal of Professional Nursing 33* (2017): 173–174. http://dx.doi.org/10.1016/j.profnurs.2017.04.003.

39. Hassmiller, Susan B. "Nursings' Role in Building a Culture of Health." In Sandra B. Lewenson & Marie Truglio-Londrigan (Eds.). *Practicing Primary Health Care in*

Nursing: Caring for Populations, 33–60. Burlington, MA: Jones & Bartlett Learning, (2017); "Black Nursing Students and Schools of Nursing," no date. Pocket Knowledge, Teachers College, Columbia University, New York, NY. http://pocketknowledge.tc.columbia.edu/home.php/viewfile/75064; Threat, Charissa J. *Nursing Civil Rights: Gender and Race in the Army Nurse Corps.* Urbana, Chicago, and Springfield, IL: University of Illinois Press, (2015); Pitt-Mosley, Marie Oleatha. *A History of Black Leaders in Nursing: The Influence of Four Black Community Health Nurses on the Establishment, Growth, and Practice of Public Health Nurses in New York City, 1900–1930* (Ed.D. diss., Teachers College, Columbia University) (1992). http://pocketknowledge.tc.columbia.edu/home.php/viewfile/8534.

40. Thoms, Adah Bell. "Greetings to the National Medical Association-Delivered by Mrs. Adah Bell Thoms, RN, at Philadelphia, August 30, 1917." *Journal of the National Medical Association* 10, no. 1 (March 1918): 52–53. https://www.ncbi.nlm.nih.gov/pmc/issues/175426/.

Sandra B. Lewenson, RN, EdD, FAAN
College of Health Professions
Lienhard School of Nursing
Pace University
Bedford Road
Pleasantville, NY 10706

ARTICLES

"Not Only with Thy Hands, But Also with Thy Minds": Salvaging Psychologically Damaged Soldiers in the Second World War

Jane Brooks
The University of Manchester

Abstract. This essay breaks new ground in exploring the tensions in female nursing during the Second World War as the mental health needs of the injured were increasingly acknowledged. Advances in weaponry and transportation meant that the Second World War was a truly global war with mobile troops and enhanced capacity to maim and kill. A critical mass of female nursing sisters was posted to provide care for physical trauma, yet the nature of this uniquely modern war also required nurses to provide psychological support for troops readying for return to action. Most nursing sisters of the British Army had little or no mental health training, but there were trained male mental health nurses available. Publications of broadcasts by the Matron-in-Chief of the British Army Nursing Service detail the belief that the female nurse was the officer in charge of the ward when the patients had physical needs. However, that the nursing sister held this position when the patients' requirements were of a psychological nature was at times tested and contested. Through personal testimony and contemporary accounts in the nursing and medical press, this essay investigates how female nursing staff negotiated their position as the expert by the psychologically damaged combatants' bedside. The essay identifies the resourcefulness of nurses to ensure access to all patient groups and also their determination to move the boundaries of their professional work to support soldiers in need.

In 1942, psychiatric nurse Fritz Schindler began an article in the *American Journal of Nursing* with a polemic for new psychiatric technologies. "The last

Nursing History Review 27 (2019): 29–56. A Publication of the American Association for the History of Nursing. Copyright © 2019 Springer Publishing Company.
http://dx.doi.org/10.1891/1062-8061.27.29

two decades have raised the treatment of the mentally ill from a custodial level to one of strict and specific therapy. The shock therapies are the most outstanding and successful type of treatment: of this group electro-shock is the newest and most widely used form."[1] He ended the article with the impassioned words, "Nurses have an entirely new role in this latest therapeutic weapon against mental disease."[2] Although he was not the only nurse to extoll the virtues of new scientific treatments for mental illness, it is perhaps no coincidence that he was a male psychiatric nurse writing about advances that could professionalize psychiatric nursing work. Shock treatments, like electroconvulsive and coma therapies were brought to British hospitals by the beginning of the Second World War. Here too they were heralded as successful treatments for psychiatric illnesses, especially schizophrenia.[3]

Not all nurses were convinced by the efficacy of these quasi-experimental therapies. American nurse Hildegard Peplau is considered to have revolutionized psychiatric nursing in the United States and in the post-war era had significant influence on Annie Altschul who was to become the first professor of psychiatric nursing in Britain. Posted to the 312th Military Hospital in England, Peplau witnessed first hand the administration of sodium amytal to induce deep coma. Convinced that this practice was "obscene," she began to lobby to be allowed to begin talking therapy for the soldiers.[4] Peplau was unusual; she was a mental-trained female nurse with a wealth of experience in caring for psychiatrically and psychologically ill patients. Few British Army nurses posted to overseas war service could boast such credentials. In the absence of mental training, they needed to rely on the knowledge of psychiatrists and mental-trained male nursing orderlies.

The purpose of this essay is to examine the tensions in the female nursing sisters' postings to military hospitals overseas to care for psychologically and psychiatrically damaged combatants.[5] The tensions bring into stark relief the challenges of shifting gender and professional boundaries on active service in the Second World War, as the Queen Alexandra's Imperial Military Nursing Service (Q.A.s) negotiated their place in frontline duties with this patient group.[6] Using a combination of personal testimony and the professional press, the essay argues that despite the majority of British nurses' lack of psychological and psychiatric training, they managed to harness their considerable nursing skills to provide suitable care. However, this was at least in part at both a gendered and professional cost. Their lack of training meant that they needed to rely on the psychiatric knowledge of their male medical colleagues and the nursing experience of male medical orderlies who had worked in mental hospitals before the war. Male nursing orderlies may have been registered mental nurses, but they were not commissioned officers like their female nursing counterparts.[7] The male mental nurses' technical skills with scientific treatments would have called into question the requirement for female nursing sisters in frontline psychiatric wards. In psychiatric military hospitals in Britain, male noncommissioned officer (NCO) mental-trained nurses deputized for the ward sister when she was off duty.[8] There may have been general acquiescence that the female nurse was the officer in charge of the ward when the patients had physical needs, but that she held this position when the patients' requirements were of a psychological nature was at times tested and contested.

The essay will begin with an overview of the status of psychiatric nursing in Britain in the first half of the 20th century. This will be followed by a discussion of the presence of female nurses on active service overseas in the Second World War, and the expectation that she would be "an officer and a lady,"[9] as well as the professional expert at the bedside. It will then consider the attitudes of the medical and nursing professions toward mental illness and the slow changes to the understanding of psychological war-damage from the First World War and into the Second. The range of treatment options will then be explored, including those instigated by the nurses themselves as part of their caring work, those sanctioned by the medical and occupational therapy professions, but invariably part of the nurse's role and those instigated by the medical profession as part of the developments in psychiatry and psychiatric science.

It is not the intention to argue that psychiatric and psychological conditions were synonymous. Literature of the time tends to differentiate between psychological problems that are brought on by the trauma of war, such as "when the peril becomes imminent,"[10] and psychiatric problems that are more long-standing such as "the schizophrenic type illness."[11] Psychiatrists were also keen to differentiate themselves from their "psychological colleagues."[12] Despite the acknowledgment of these differences, the two areas of practice were clearly inter-related and treatment regimens for men with both serious psychiatric illnesses and the more transitory psychological trauma associated with battle-exhaustion were to some extent interchangeable.[13] Furthermore, as Peter Nolan and Niall McCrae argue, in the period just prior to the Second World War, psychiatry was still "commonly known in Britain as psychological medicine."[14]

"You Were Prepared to Do Your Training [and] that Was Good Enough."[15]

The nursing sisters of the British Army who went to war between 1939 and 1945 were all women and all had trained within the general hospital apprenticeship system.[16] Few had experienced the care of psychiatrically ill or psychologically damaged patients. Only women on the General State Register[17] were entitled to join the Q.A.s, so even the very few psychiatrically trained nursing sisters available, also needed to be State Registered Nurses (SRN).[18] To qualify for both registers could take up to 6 years.[19] Given that nursing imposed a marriage bar until the middle years of the war and was for most "a short-term expedient before marriage," for many this would not have been an attractive option.[20] Nursing care on hospital wards was located in the physical needs of the patient and those in charge expected a professional that is, "impersonal" relationship with patients.[21] The nurses' day was routine and regimented in line with the needs of the honorary medical staff, hospital service and the demands of the senior nurses who needed to provide safe care for patients with a largely student workforce.[22]

According to the demands of the hospital "machine" and the ideology of female nurses' deference to masculine authority, the nurses of the Second World War had been trained to function in a female profession in a male profession's world.[23] Their registration to practice was sanctioned through the male-dominated parliament and their work was sanctioned by the male-dominated medical profession.[24] Despite the overall power lying within the male hegemony, British general nurses' registration was at least nominally regulated through the General Nursing Council, a predominantly female organization.[25] Until 1951, nurses in psychiatric hospitals could also be examined through the Medico-Psychological Association (MPA), run by and for psychiatrists. In 1927, The Lancet proclaimed that the GNC examinations were too costly and set at "too high a standard in general nursing for those who only wish to register as mental nurses,"[26] suggesting that even psychiatrists thought mental nurses were of a lower ability than their general nursing colleagues.[27] Whether those who chose to enter mental nursing were necessarily less academically able is not clear. There is evidence, however that the entry criteria were not always so stringent. Sister Cecelia Christie started her psychiatric training at the age of 16 years old. Although the official starting age was 18 years old, they did not ask to see any documents. In her oral history she maintained that, "the very fact that you were prepared to do your training ... was good enough."[28] Maybe because Christie had started her mental training so young, she was willing to follow it with her general nursing. Once qualified in both mental and general nursing, Christie became a valuable and unusual asset. She was eventually sent with the advance 32 psychiatric unit into Normandy.[29]

The control of the MPA lay firmly in the hands of the male medical profession. According to Claire Chatterton, doctors were convinced that mental nurses should be ruled by doctors,[30] because "their fellow-nurses still tended to despise them."[31] The MPA curriculum was dictated by the medical profession and only doctors could examine for it. Into the 1920s, some institutions gave precedence to the MPA qualification over the GNC, though others did understand the benefits of the nursing profession's own examination and registration.[32] If the professional boundaries between medicine, mental nursing, and general nursing were in conflict, the gender and class issues only fuelled difficulties. While general nursing was almost entirely female, men had traditionally been part of the mental nursing workforce and tended to be of a lower socioeconomic class to their female general nurse colleagues.[33]

Psychiatric nursing did not form part of the general nurse training curriculum until late in the 20th century and psychiatric training was not as popular a profession for women as general nursing. Few general nurses had any experience or knowledge of the work of their mental nursing colleagues, adding to the general distrust.[34] Ironically however, British mental nurses were much closer to their general nursing colleagues than to their psychiatrically trained colleagues from the United States. If Peplau and her compatriots' training was grounded in modern ideas of therapeutic relationships,[35] their British counterparts were more likely to emulate the impersonal regimens of the general hospital. John Adams refers to the ubiquity of nurses' engagement with physical treatments rather than psychological care in some British hospitals until the 1950s.[36] In the 1930s, against the growing unionisation of male mental nurses, the number of female recruits into mental nursing declined.[37] Chris Hart argues that this loss of women and perhaps most particularly women of a higher social class led to a rising conservatism in mental health,[38] and what Tommy Dickinson and colleagues describe as a desire to "carry out the orders of the medical staff or their nursing superiors uncritically and without question."[39] It was out of these disparate grouping of occupational alignments that nurses who would salvage psychologically damaged men in the Second World War arose.

Women's Place in the Second World War

Female nursing sisters' access to the men sick in mind near the frontline was dependent upon a complex brokering of their general skills as nurses and their womanhood. Penny Summerfield and Corinna Peniston-Bird argue, "The Second World War was one of the most contradictory periods in British history for the boundary between male and female roles."[40] In some respects, it was a more gender inclusive time than other periods and other wars.[41] It was the first war into which women were conscripted.[42] Women war workers wore trousers like their male counterparts, thus blurring the boundaries of gender difference.[43] Women undertook a range of often dangerous war-work on the home front including fire watching and working anti-aircraft batteries. Nurse Betty Crisp recalled fire watching with a stirrup pump from the pathology laboratory at her training hospital after a day on the wards.[44] The decision that young single women should be conscripted to work where they were needed, irrespective of the distance they would need to travel from home, significantly lessened long-held ideas about supervision and chaperonage.[45] Nurse Margaret Parkes who trained at Addenbrookes Hospital in Cambridge maintained that:

> They [hospital authorities] were afraid of them leading the sort of life their parents wouldn't approve of … and the war changed all that … and during my time I saw that attitude change … society changed and everybody was taking risks. Before it was a protective culture, of girls particularly. I mean when people are in Ack Ack [anti-aircraft] units, you're not going to worry about when they go out at night in Cambridge.[46]

Nevertheless, much of the work that women undertook as part of the war effort continued to be gendered.[47] Women could build guns, maintain them, even aim them, but they were not allowed to fire them.[48] When women engaged in dangerous activities on overseas service, such as espionage, their "femaleness" was crucial to that work.[49] As Juliette Pattinson argues, female members of the Special Operations Executive, "endeavour[s] not to reveal themselves as clandestine agents while operational were often accomplished through performances of hyper-femininity."[50] The gendered contradictions of war service prevailed for all women war workers and nurses on overseas duty were no different to their "sisters" in factories and offices in Britain. Even if they could circumvent those contradictions through parlaying their clinical nursing skills with the physically ill or injured combatant, access to psychologically damaged men made the contradictions more obvious. There was apparently little reason for their presence over male psychiatrically trained nurses, except their femininity.

Nursing Work and Nurses' Presence

Advances in transport and weapon technologies since the First World War meant that any following wars would be more mobile and troops better equipped to kill and maim.[51] Developments in land, sea and airborne transport enabled mass mobilization of forces into hostile environments such as the deserts of the Middle East and North Africa and the jungles of Burma and India. Nevertheless, although hitherto isolated places were now accessible to allied troops, there remained significant difficulties in transporting men rapidly away from such areas for medical treatments. Having demonstrated their value in caring for ill and injured soldiers during the First World War,[52] the use of Q.A.s in this new conflict was understood as crucial for the success of the Army Medical Services. Despite the often unwelcomed wholesale "intrusion of women into what clearly should be the one impregnable male bastion,"[53] for the first time a critical mass of female nurses were posted into far-flung and dangerous war zones to care for the troops.

In March 1944, an officer who had been fighting at the Anzio beachhead wrote to his wife of the impact of the nursing sisters in comparison with the orderlies of the Royal Army Medical Corps (RAMC). The letter was reprinted in *The Nursing Times*, later in the year:

> But what is this! these [sic] funny figures in battle dress cannot be R.A.M.C. orderlies (and a woman in battle dress can look funny), God bless 'em the Q.A.s are here! Our own women are with us. Up go the drooping tails! they [sic] must not see how near we were to the dread-edge of panic! They're taking it too!... the sickly smell of blood, the bravely stifled groan, the dim lights—only a Hogarth could paint it, a Rupert Brooke sing it, the magnificent epic defiance of these women. What a tribute to the discipline of a hospital training. Now this does not one whit detract from our men of the R.A.M.C. I have been deeply moved at the tenderness of a man to a man, but the QAs bring more than tenderness. No more strategically intelligent order was ever given than to send the QAs to the beachhead. The morale of a desperate venture was injected with a new vitality.[54]

It was not that men who worked in a nursing capacity were rough or uncaring, it was that the female nurses' presence both calmed the men who were too ill to fight and also created an environment in which men's morale was raised. According to Kara Dixon Vuic, even 20 years later during the Vietnam War, recruitment campaigns for military nursing used the femininity of the nurse rather than her clinical skills as the method of patient healing.[55] Yet, during the Second World War, rhetoric of the nursing sisters' presence being important because of their gender, needs to be tempered with the reality that no other women were allowed to go into frontline areas. When postings to overseas duties were expanded to other female members of the military following the D-Day landings in 1944, they were retained in base units away from the fighting,[56] while the nurses got closer. In 1944, nursing sisters were posted to the Anzio beachhead as the war raged around and above them.[57] Sister Penny Salter and her colleagues were posted to a field hospital in Death Valley on the Burma Road to care for an outbreak of scrub typhus.

Nursing may have been considered the epitome of feminine work and the most appropriate war work for women,[58] yet paradoxically nurses were often the only women allowed in the masculine space of a war zone, subverting the "contract" that men make to defend them.[59] The long-held belief that the purpose of war was to protect women, meant that not all in the military supported the posting of women into dangerous places: "the front is understood as a place where women are not."[60] As Cynthia Enloe remarked, what military commanders wanted from nurses was simply not compatible. They wanted nurses as women to perform their natural caring skills to support soldiers' healing, but how could they be "enlisted as military nurses if, as 'women,' they are supposed to be excluded from the 'front.'"[61] In her war, diary Sister Mary Morris described the troops attitude to the nurses' "temerity in entering this 'man's' world," as they waited for their landing orders off the Normandy coast in June 1944.[62] Despite such attitudes female nurses' skills were needed close to the frontline, female military nurses were essential in combat zones to salvage combatants, partly because they were women and partly because they were skilled providers of care and technical treatments.[63]

British nursing sisters' hospital training had prepared them for the physical care they would need to provide for their combatant patients. As student nurses their duties had been physically demanding over long hours, often within hierarchical regimes that were themselves harsh and unyielding: "she [the student nurse] will realise that her training is steadily conditioning her whole personality to undertake hard, responsible and vitally important work."[64] Writing in her diary after arriving in Normandy shortly after D-Day, Sister Ann Radloff stated, "This was the moment for which I had prepared for four long years."[65] Sister Brenda McBryde's memories following her landing in Normandy in June 1944 were that, "Everything I had learned during four hard years of training suddenly made sense. My hands had a sure and certain skill and my brain was unflustered as I replaced dressings over gaping wounds, gave injections of morphia and the new wonder drug, penicillin, charted blood pressures."[66]

Much of the nurses' work would have been to recover the broken bodies of men and nurses' skills were needed despite the ideological difficulties their presence created.[67] However, the "uniquely modern form of warfare" that epitomised the global machine of the Second World War, also demanded that nurses engaged in managing the emotions of combatants and healing their minds ready to return them to fight.[68] The limitations in the nursing sisters' knowledge and skills with psychologically damaged men meant their presence to care for this patient group was more difficult to explain. A decision to use trained male mental nurses in frontline duties to care for psychiatrically and psychologically damaged men, rather than general trained female nursing officers would have been more in line with gender attitudes.

Male psychiatrically trained nurses in the 1940s were in the RAMC, not the Q.A.s and were not "nursing officers, equal in every way to the female nursing officer."[69] Yet, the presence of these trained men on overseas service, even if they were deployed in the other ranks,[70] raise questions regarding the decision to post female nursing sisters not trained in psychiatry to forward areas. Given the limited training of female nurses in psychological care, it is unclear what skills they had that were so necessary as to defy an ideology that demanded "protection" and instead were posted to highly dangerous front-line duties to care for this patient group. According to F.A.E. Crew, who had not only served in the war, but was later the official medical historian of the war, "although male and female nurses can be completely equal in respect of professional knowledge and skill they still remain distinct for one is male and the other female. The difference would seem of considerable importance in so far as nursing is concerned."[71] Twenty-three years after the end of the Second World War, the continued importance of a nurse's presence as a "mother-figure, tender and compassionate [was seen to] advantage the patient greatly."[72] Military commanders were aware that female nurses were a powerful tool in "lifting the lonely soldier's morale,"[73] essential if psychologically damaged men were to be returned to battle.

The judgment not to use trained male nurses was constructed predominantly through arguments of the value of women's presence to the war effort. Female nurses were caught in a liminal position in which rather than their clinical skills giving them access to troops, it was their womanhood. Whether or not they understood their role with psychologically and psychiatrically damaged soldiers in this way is not known. Once with this patient group, they used their resourcefulness to ensure their continued place as the expert at the bedside. As the war progressed and psychological trauma lost some of its stigma, nurses made legitimate claims about the healing value of compassion in order to access the sick in mind. Paradoxically, given the potential dangers of new psychiatric treatments, they were also able to negotiate their presence because this work required physical nursing, if some of the more experimental regimes were not to cause pathological damage to the men.

Attitudes to Mental Illness

Between the First and Second World Wars, there were slow and uneven shifts in the understanding of mental illness caused by war, shifts that can be seen through an increasingly sympathetic nomenclature. In the First World

War, the term "shell-shock" was developed to describe, "distress caused by the participation—or the anticipation of—combat."[74] The role of the nurse as one who could, "offer patients not just the chance to survive, but also the reasons to live," was critical to supporting men suffering from shell-shock.[75] Nevertheless, suspicions around mental illness remained. In 1941, an article in *The Lancet* maintained that many of those who presented with psychological trauma caused by war were considered to be "scrimshanker[s]… who feel that they must bolster up their illness with adventitious aid."[76] Mental illness brought on by battle still had a reputation as a popular complaint, as it was more difficult to determine than physical illnesses or injuries and led to decent pensions.[77] "Malingering" was still conceived as a real possibility among men,[78] and nursing staff still held a broad range of attitudes to mental illness. In her diary for July 27, 1942, Sister Nell Jarrett was critical of the overly kind organization of psychiatric care for prisoners of war. She acknowledged the belief of the medical officer Mac, with whom she worked, who "says lots recover with a rest. Lots more are malingerers."[79]

"Lack of Moral Fibre (LMF)" was first introduced in 1940 as an administrative term by the Air Ministry, rather than a psychiatric diagnosis. According to Edgar Jones, its purpose was to deter aircrew from refusing to fly.[80] Along with "not yet diagnosed nervous" (NYDN), it soon predominated and by the early years of the desert war in 1941, was part of a repertoire of diagnoses.[81] By 1942, doctors were starting to believe that acute neurotic symptoms could be brought on by battle exhaustion as well as predisposing factors related to upbringing and heredity.[82] If it was an extensive duration of combat that could create such psychological trauma,[83] then these men could be rehabilitated relatively easily by removing them from battle. The work of the nurses in encouraging participation in rehabilitation became an important part of their role, in which they could "help a great deal by making sure that everyone possible attends [occupational therapy], and by taking an interest in the patients' work."[84] Notwithstanding the movement toward a more sympathetic attitude, the understanding of mental illness still lagged behind that of physical medicine.

In the wake of the First World War, changing attitudes toward the inevitability of shell-shock among combatants led to the number of military psychiatrists being drastically reduced.[85] If fewer soldiers would in future succumb to shell shock, because of improved selection practices, fewer psychiatrists would be needed.[86] This conviction however belied the reality that in order to prevent the mentally unfit from active service, selection would need to occur. There was a general acknowledgment that testing for physical illness was becoming increasingly sophisticated, but better psychiatric testing was still needed to prevent the mentally unfit from finding their way into the Army.[87] According to Edgar Jones, in 1939 there were only about six regular medical officers with psychiatric training.[88] Such woefully low numbers would stymie successful selection in the early years of the war. It was not until the third year of war that accepted techniques for determining the best recruits were appropriately employed by the Army.[89]

The majority of the medical staff were unsure of how to treat the men damaged by war. An article in *The Lancet* in 1944 argued that, "It is a sad reflection on medical education to find that the combatant officer often has a better understanding of such cases and may be more effective in their handling than many medical men."[90] The need to rehabilitate the psychologically damaged was crucial in all theaters of war, given the percentage of soldiers—put at between 10% and 30% of all sick and wounded men evacuated from battle zones—who succumbed to battle-exhaustion and more complex psychiatric conditions.[91] Army Rest Centres were set up close to the frontline to provide rapid treatment for those with a diagnosis of battle exhaustion and then be able return men to battle as quickly as possible on recovery.[92] There was an appreciation that not all men who suffered from psychological damage were simply exhausted and those with more serious problems were removed further away from the battle zones. These policies, as ambitious as they were, were also flawed. Although it was believed that most men would return to battle fitness, the actual figures were far lower. The percentage of soldiers able to return to combat duty varied between different theaters of war, but it was generally about 20%, the rest were either invalided back home, or returned to non-combat duties,[93] far more kindly outcomes than returning men psychologically damaged by war back to battle.

For all patients, this increased sympathy and pathologizing, rather than stigmatizing required additional beds to be made available in frontline areas as well as base hospitals away from the front and the beds needed nursing staff.[94] Successful care of psychologically damaged men, including those with psychiatric illness required a blurring of doctor, nurse, and patient boundaries. The development of "therapeutic communities" was an important aspect of this new type of care, but such novel regimes did not necessarily foster the total removal of hierarchies.[95] If the numbers of psychiatrically trained doctors with whom the nurses worked rose during the war, the care of the psychologically damaged soldier were still often left to the most inexperienced doctors, and those from the then colonies.[96] Captain Biswas, the Indian medical officer in charge of mentally ill patients on the hospital ship on which Sister Catherine Hutchinson worked was also the most junior doctor on board: "I asked Biswas if he had been taught anything about mental illness in his training. 'Not a thing!' he said cheerfully, 'but the orderlies have all worked in mental hospitals, and have ways of calming patients.' One was, he told me was to give them an enema."[97]

Hutchinson does not state what she thinks of this treatment, though the impression is that she did not consider it appropriate. It is also possible that as a white European, she found being placed under the authority of an Indian doctor difficult. Making him appear less than competent could have been a method of reducing the specter of what she saw as an unfortunate position. Mostly the nursing staff appeared to believe that the use of compassion in their nursing was the only beneficial treatment option. As one Canadian nursing sister described, "You just had to let them do the talking."[98] It was a type of nursing that was in many ways at odds with the regimented work of the hospital nurse, it required "infinite tact and patience but it is very worthwhile."[99]

"Now I Am Safe from Harm": Female Nurses and Thoughtful Care

On September 16, 1939, *The Nursing Mirror* published an article by the psychiatrist Charles Stanford Read: "The nurse and the psychological emergencies of war." The article sought to prepare nurses for the emergency admission of patients who were suffering from "war-scare" or "nerve shock," to a first aid unit, or hospital.[100] The most important role of the nurse according to Stanford Read was:

> by her understanding, sympathetic and calm attitude may bring a large measure of mental peace and instil much of that feeling. "Now I am safe from harm." It is largely the child within us that makes us afraid. To her terrified patient the nurse assumes the role of a mother.[101]

If to the modern reader, the sublimation of a clinical nurse's skills into the task of mothering appears to lessen their significant talents in recovering their patients, there is little to suggest that the nurses in the Second World War saw it in the same way. In October 1943, Sister Agnes Morgan wrote to her mother about one 19-year-old soldier who told her, "me [*sic*] mother makes OXO for me when I feel sick at home."[102] Sister Francie Brown wrote to her family of a particularly nervous patient who, "depended on me absolutely."[103] In her oral history interview, Sister Emily Soper spoke of a nurse colleague who cared for two young German prisoners of war: "And they were both crying for their mothers. And my friend had two, had twin brothers of 16 at home in Yorkshire, so she took these two boys in her arms to comfort them, because that is what she hoped someone would do to her brothers."[104] Morris recalled a young officer who had been wounded at the Battle of Arnhem:

> He was wounded after 8 days of hell, no food just some fruit from the Dutch civilians—very little water and no sleep. Men were running around screaming, trying to find any escape. He was taken to a Dutch hospital behind German lines. He had two abdominal operations performed by a German surgeon and was well cared for by Dutch nurses. B--- will be alright physically once the wound has healed but I think it will be a long time before he gets over the shock of Arnhem. Connie tells me that he had to be constantly sedated at night to stop him screaming in terror. He is only 22 years old.[105]

Soper's concerns were for the men in France with self-inflicted wounds:

> We could see why, for some of these young men it was a trauma … the whole war was a trauma for them and you could understand why they had tried to cause a self-inflicted wound, which was usually in the foot.[106]

It is clear from these vignettes that the nursing sisters of the Second World War felt that their patients should be treated with sympathy and kind-heartedness. The language they used suggests they understood the importance of providing the security of a domestic arrangement, in which the nurse is the mother in the tripartite relationship between the father/doctor, mother/nurse, and patient/child.[107] According to Evelyn Pearce in her 1937 edition of *A General Textbook of Nursing*, a nurse's role was to provide an environment that is "free from fear, inspires confidence and provides an atmosphere of peace, serenity and security which is so important an adjunct to the relaxation of mind and body necessary for recovery from disease."[108]

In a report on psychiatric medicine in 1943, G.W.B. James, a consultant in psychological medicine, reflected that the nursing staff assigned to psychiatric hospitals gave excellent care and were clinically competent, yet "a number never really liked nursing in a psychiatric unit."[109] One Territorial Army Nursing Sister (TANS) attached to No. 1 Psychiatric Hospital in the Middle East admitted that the care of psychiatric patients was, "theoretically absorbing and highly interesting, but practically depressing and trying."[110] Nevertheless, she stated, "I learnt more about humanity and the multiple small and great troubles of mankind than I had learnt in any 10 years of my life before."[111] James offers no explanation for the assumptions he made regarding nurses' attitudes to caring for men who were sick in mind. It may be that some did not like the work. The work was so different to nursing in a general hospital in peacetime and psychiatric nursing was not generally well considered. Yet, the personal testimonies do not bear out his opinions. British nursing sisters may have discussed the care they proffered for psychologically damaged men less than they did for those with physical injuries.[112] They may even have found the work harder; Morgan voiced her concerns in a letter to her mother about her abilities in this area.[113] Nevertheless, their descriptions identify kindness, thoughtfulness, and a willingness to test professional boundaries in order to support recovery. They may have parlayed their womanhood and particularly their motherly attributes to gain access to psychologically damaged men, but it is clear that their empathy and compassion had a significant impact on the treatment regimens.

The Second World War witnessed a growing acknowledgment that even the best soldiers could succumb to mental distress[114] and there was a softening toward mental health problems in the Army as the war progressed.[115] But not all medical staff supported the more kindly and motherly treatment of the nurses. When doctors' clinical distance collided with nurses' compassion in a unit where the doctors assumed complete control, it was difficult for nurses to manage. Even in more egalitarian working environments professional relationships could be stressed to their limit. Nurses learnt to differentiate between those patients who were anxious and needed to talk, those who were "mentally deficient [and] transferred to the Pioneer Corps,"[116] and those who "were really old neurotics who simply lived on our kindness and sympathy."[117] But their assessment of patient-type was not always supported by the doctor in charge of the unit. Morris was particularly critical of the medical officer in her hospital who considered one young officer to be "swinging the lead." Morris' diary states that whilst she believes this medical officer was "kind and competent in dealing with the physically injured. Why can he not see that the mind of this sensitive man has been shattered by the horrors he has seen here in Normandy?"[118] Morris expressed her frustration at not being able to send her patient back to England.

In order to circumvent some of the potential harshness of the regime, while maintaining the vision of dutiful obedience to the male military machine, Morris quietly used unorthodox methods to support her psychologically damaged patients. Her chief practice was to involve patients in each other's care: "Their interest and warmth will be [the] best therapy here."[119] Such thoughtful care would she hoped encourage her psychiatrically ill patients to recover. Later she acknowledged "how delighted the men are to be given information about their own case history and treatment. It gives them a feeling of involvement."[120] Such openness of treatment regimens also gave other patients a sense of purpose and to put them once again in charge of their own and their colleagues' lives. Morris remained aware that her ward organization may not have been positively viewed by her superiors,[121] but its efficacy was similar to more mainstream occupational therapy; the patients started to feel useful once more and thus perhaps better able to return to battle.

Occupational Therapy

For patients and their nurses, one of the most prevalent official forms of treatment for battle exhaustion was occupational therapy.[122] Occupational therapy had been used to support the rehabilitation of the mentally ill since the 19th century. Unlike the relatively new innovations in physiotherapy,[123] active rehabilitation through farming, gardening, and domestic physical labor not only provided economic stability to asylums, but could also help develop a sense of usefulness in patients.[124] The value of occupational therapy as a treatment for combatants was established in the First World War, with nurses and specially trained women undertaking a variety of activities with wounded and psychologically damaged men.[125] Ana Carden-Coyne suggests that in this earlier war there was a gradation from craft activities, such as basket-weaving, book-binding, leather work, and sign-writing that were heavily supported by the Red Cross, to more manly pursuits such as industrial work or gardening.[126] Craft work was occasionally disparaged as were the women who promoted it.[127] However, although there were some who considered basket weaving and needlework demeaning for a soldier, for men who had been feminized by their mental breakdown,[128] it was a method of starting to reaffirm their abilities before they returned to battle. Sister I.B.H., who worked in a psychiatric hospital for officers, believed that once the men "settle[s] down to constructing a variety of things and taking a pride in doing so" the scorn for such activities lessened.[129]

If the craft activities were possibly demeaning, the testimonies suggest that creating gardens both of flowers and more beneficially vegetables, were enjoyed and seen as proper work.[130] Sister Elsie Driver, having been posted to the Psychiatrical Neurological Unit in the desert, was impressed by the gardens her patients created and by the "competition [that] was great between each ward, and one can well imagine what this meant, when all around stretched miles of desert."[131] It was work that gave the men a new sense of purpose. Cynthia Toman argues that the Canadian nurses struggled at first to see occupational and social activities as nursing work at all, but they did not doubt its efficacy for mental health problems.[132] There is no evidence that the nurses reflected on the inappropriateness of occupational therapy for mentally ill soldiers. Any discussions in the nursing press or personal testimonies suggest they saw it as beneficial. An article in 1943 on "Modern mental treatment" in *The Nursing Times*, maintained: "Occupational therapy plays a large part and with physical training, organized games and swimming the patients' minds become atuned [*sic*] to normality."[133] More problematic for the demands by many female nurses that these patients should receive compassionate treatment were the range of invasive therapies given to some psychologically damaged men.

"The Necessity For a Special Nurse."[134]

Driver wrote to Dame Katharine Jones, the Matron-in-Chief of the Q.A.s that only about half of all sisters in her hospital were trained for "mental work."[135] However, she felt that this enabled them to "learn from the bottom War Neurosis."[136] Their active service training in mental nursing was supported by the "very able and helpful medical officers, who helped us considerably over a period when we felt "out of things" and taught us fully the meaning of 'Not only with thy hands but with thy mind.'"[137] In the 1940 publication, *War-time Nurse*, Angus MacNiven, the medical superintendent of the Glasgow Royal Mental Hospital maintained that, "there is no drug or medical or surgical procedure which will eradicate neurotic or psychotic symptoms ... If through her [the nurse's] conversation and her behaviour the patient comes to regard her as a source of comfort, strength, sympathy and understanding, she will help him to recover from his illness."[138] There may have been an acceptance of the importance of the kindly nurse and that there was nothing in scientific psychiatric medicine that could cure mental illness, but that did not mean that psychiatrists did not experiment with therapies or that nurses did not support them. Indeed, nurses' expertise in monitoring physically ill patients meant she was a vital adjunct to the success of such therapies and the prevention of irreversible damage.[139] In her article to *The Nursing Times* in 1944, Sister I.B.H. wrote:

> From the nursing point of view we are very fortunate in that we take in this hospital all types of mental and nervous diseases, so that we have the opportunity of dealing with a wide variety of illnesses and of using various kinds of special treatment, such as insulin shock therapy, electric shock therapy, prolonged narcosis, inductotherm and pentothal.[140]

A range of quasi-experimental treatments for mental illness, including deep coma (insulin) therapy, narcosis therapy, and electroconvulsive therapy (ECT) had been developed in the interwar period. These scientific psychiatric treatments provided general trained nurses with a legitimate claim for access to psychologically damaged patients. Paradoxically however, these treatments placed the nurses very much as the assistant of the doctor. For some nurses, the therapies were the antithesis of the gentle compassionate nursing many felt the men needed. Nevertheless, not all showed antipathy toward them.[141] In some cases, their acceptance of some of the more invasive and dangerous therapies highlights their relative acquiescence to danger in the face of potential personal and professional development that access to scientific medicine could offer. For many nurses, the engagement with these technologies was entirely new and was seen as vindication of their professional abilities. Coma therapies of various descriptions and shock therapy required skilled monitoring of the patient's vital signs, nutrition needed to be carefully reintroduced following insulin coma therapy and acute restlessness after the induction of hyperpyrexia required vigilant management. In an article to the *Journal of Neurology, Neurosurgery & Psychiatry* in 1939, R.D. Gillespie argued that in order for the necessary "rapport" to be achieved and thus render the treatment successful, it was necessary to have a "special nurse" for the day.[142] As I.B.H. maintained:

> Prolonged narcosis is given for anxiety states with considerable agitation, or for depressive or manic states where electric convulsion is for some reason contra-indicated. By the use of special drugs the patient is kept asleep as long as possible during the 24 hours. This treatment is continues for 14 days or more, during which time very careful nursing is required.[143]

One TANS sister wrote of the "very interesting cases who had special treatment, occasionally the psychiatrist cured a patient in a way which seemed quite miraculous."[144] Whilst she did not specify the treatment, it is clear from the letter to Dame Katharine Jones that it was not the normal talking therapy. I.B.H. discussed the use of pentothal to relax patients in order for them to engage in psychotherapy and the use of "hyperpyrexia by inductotherm ... for cases of general paralysis of the insane," an alternative treatment at the time to malarial therapy.[145] Although these treatments were potentially dangerous, some had effected improvements if not cures in some patients.[146] Even the possibility of their efficacy meant that some nurses were keen to be part of what was heralded in the medical press as a "therapeutic team,"[147] a term probably used by psychiatrists to foster allegiances, as much as to describe any truly inter-professional mode of working.

Conclusion

War was considered a masculine space, which made the posting of women into areas close to the fighting problematic.[148] Nevertheless, female nurses had made claims for access to ill and injured combatants from the Crimean War in the mid-19th century. By the Second World War, the nursing sisters of the British Army and other allied forces were being posted to far-flung places to recover men for return to battle or to rescue them for non-combatant duties. Whilst there were some at the highest level of military authority—including General Bernard Montgomery whose 8th Army fought and defeated Field Marshall Erwin Rommel's German Africa Corps in the desert war, 1941–1943[149]—who were keen for nurses to be sent on active service overseas, the posting of female nurses to forward areas was not without its detractors.[150] Nurses were required to enter into careful negotiations for access to ill and injured men at the frontline, which included acknowledging their presence as women, to boost the "morale" of the troops,[151] and also their clinical nursing skills. These negotiations faced additional difficulties when the care to be proffered was to men who were psychologically rather than physically damaged, as few female nurses had psychiatric training. There were mental-trained male orderlies to care for these patients. Yet, the female nurses were given the responsibility for the care of psychologically damaged troops.

In the absence of psychiatric training, the nursing sisters used their femininity to facilitate their access combatant patients. Once with the patients they demonstrated a resourcefulness to make themselves invaluable and demonstrate their ability to learn quickly the needs of the psychologically damaged soldier. However, this created an additional layer of complexity to their position and demands they be understood as the expert by the bedside. In order to gain the required knowledge, they needed to learn psychiatric nursing skills from male mental-trained orderlies and clinical psychiatric knowledge from the medical officers. The negotiations were compounded by the value of their physical nursing skills with patients undergoing quasi-experimental and potentially dangerous therapies and their participation in them. Arguably however, the most influential of their care practices with these patients was their unique understanding of compassionate care that they had gathered through their encounters with combatants during the conflict. It was this and their willingness to use their minds to care for this patient group that supported the recovery of men emotionally damaged by war.

Acknowledgments

I am grateful to the Queen Alexandra's Royal Army Nursing Corps Association for supporting the project on British Army in the Second World War Army.

Notes

1. Fritz H. Schindler, "Nursing in Electro-Shock Therapy," *American Journal of Nursing 42*, no. 8 (1942): 858.
2. Schindler, "Nursing in Electro-Shock Therapy," 861.
3. John Adams, "The Nursing Role in the Use of Insulin Coma Therapy for Schizophrenia in Britain, (1936–1965)," *Journal of Advanced Nursing 70*, no. 9 (2014): 2086–94.
4. For a full and detailed analysis of Peplau's life and work see, Barbara J. Callaway, *Hildegard Peplau: Psychiatric Nurse of the Century* (New York: Springer Publishing Co., 2002).
5. Even after the female nurses of the Queen Alexandra's Imperial Military Nursing Service (Q.A.s) were given commissioned officer status in 1941, they continued to carry the title "Sister," rather than "Lieutenant," "Captain" etc. In keeping with the nomenclature of the Second World War, this essay will refer to those female nurses who served with the Q.A.s as "Sister" or "Nursing Sister." The term "Nurse" will be used for all other registered nurses and nursing students.
6. For a thorough analysis of the professional, practice, and gender negotiations entered into by British Army nurses in the Second World War to create a place for themselves on the frontline, see, Jane Brooks, *Negotiating Nursing: British Army Sisters and Soldiers in the Second World War* (Manchester: Manchester University Press, forthcoming 2018).
7. F.A.E. Crew, "The Army Medical Services," in *Medical Services in War: The Principal Medical Lessons of the Second World War*, ed. Arthur Salusbury MacNalty, & W. Franklin Mellor (London: Her Majesty's Stationery Office (hereafter HMSO), 1968), 80.
8. I.B.H. "In Step with The Q.A.s. 2. – Nursing in a Psychiatric Hospital for Officers," *Nursing Times* (August 12, 1944): 557.
9. Cynthia Toman, *An Officer and a Lady: Canadian Military Nursing and the Second World War* (Vancouver: University of British Columbia Press, 2007).
10. Charles Stanford Read, "The Nurse and the Psychological Emergencies of War," *Nursing Mirror* (September 16, 1939): 319.
11. I.B.H. "In Step with the Q.A.s. 2. – Nursing in a Psychiatric Hospital for Officers," *Nursing Times* (August 12, 1944): 557.
12. G.W.B. James, "Psychiatric Lessons from Active Service," *The Lancet* (December 22, 1945): 802.
13. Anonymous, "Psychiatric Casualties in Battle," *The Lancet* (April 15, 1944): 505; Anonymous, "Nursing in a Psychiatric Hospital for Officers," Museum of Military Medicine (MMM) uncatalogued archive.
14. Peter Nolan and Niall McCrae, *The Story of Nursing in British Hospitals: Echoes from the Corridors* (London: Routledge, 2016), 108.
15. Cecelia Helen Burnette Christie interview by Conrad Wood, (March 25, 1993), interview 13121, Imperial War Museum (IWM) Sound Archive.

16. Mental nurse and general nurse training were completely separate in Britain at this time. Mental nurses would not have spent time during their training in a general hospital and general nurses would not have "rotated" into a mental hospital. When the author of this essay was a student nurse in the mid-1980s, it was a requirement for both mental- and general-trained nurses to have experience of each other's patient group. This is again no longer the case. The British nursing profession has always and continues to maintain separate "Fields" of practice, adult (general), child and young people, mental health, and learning disability. There is no generic training.

17. British nurses achieved the right to self-regulate in 1919 after a 30 year "battle" for nurse registration. With this right, the title "Registered Nurse," became a protected one. Only those nurses who had received a 3-year training in a general hospital were placed on the General Nursing Register. Those who had been trained in psychiatric hospitals, fever hospitals, and in sick children's nursing were placed on "Supplementary Registers" that were neither as prestigious, nor did they give the same access to senior positions in the profession. See, for example, Robert Dingwall, Anne Marie Rafferty & Charles Webster, *An Introduction to the Social History of Nursing* (London: Routledge, 1988); Susan McGann, *The Battle of the Nurses: A Study of Eight Women Who Influenced the Development of Professional Nursing,* (1880–1930) (London: Scutari Press, 1992); Monica E. Baly, *Nursing and Social Change* (London: Routledge, 1995); Anne Marie Rafferty, *The Politics of Nursing Knowledge* (London: Routledge, 1996).

18. Dame Katharine Jones, "Broadcast Talk to North America," *The British Journal of Nursing,* (November 1943): 124.

19. Rafferty, *The Politics of Nursing Knowledge,* 151.

20. Susan McGann, Anne Crowther, & Rona Dougall, *A History of the Royal College of Nursing: A Voice for Nursing, 1916–1990* (Manchester: Manchester University Press, 2009), 2.

21. Beth Linker, *War's Waste: Rehabilitation in World War I America* (Chicago, IL: University of Chicago Press, 2011).

22. For a detailed discussion of the requirements of regimentation to prevent infections at time before the availability of penicillin, see David Justham, "'Those Maggots—They Did a Wonderful Job': The Nurses' Role in Wound Management in Civilian Hospitals During the Second World War," in *One Hundred Years of Nursing Wartime Practices,* (1854–1953), eds. Jane Brooks, & Christine E. Hallett (Manchester: Manchester University Press, 2015).

23. Helen M. Sweet, & Rona Dougall, *Community Nursing and Primary Healthcare in Twentieth-Century Britain* (New York: Routledge, 2008), 36.

24. Sweet & Dougall, *Community Nursing and Primary Healthcare,* 36.

25. The General Nursing Council (GNC) was formed following the Nurses' Registration Act 1919, to compile and administer the register of qualified nurses and to approve nurse training schools attached to hospitals. For detailed discussions of the formation and problems faced by the GNC in the early to mid-20th century, see, Baly, *Nursing and Social Change*; Rafferty, *The Politics of Nursing Knowledge,* McGann et al, *A History of the Royal College of Nursing.*

26. Anonymous, "The Status of Mental Nurses," *The Lancet* (December 10, 1927): 1248.

27. The terminology for nurses in psychiatric care has changed over the years. Originally they were called keepers; their role aligned to maintaining order rather than engaging

in any sort of therapeutic endeavour (Nolan & McCrae, 7). With the Lunacy Act 1845 and the establishment of the asylum system, the term, "attendant" became the norm, though according to Peter Nolan, "these attendants were not looking for a career in the asylums, but rather a job that offered reasonable working conditions during the winter months" (1995, 252). By the end of the 19th century, "attendant" continued to be used for the male staff, but increasingly "nurse" was used for female staff (Nolan & McCrae, 53). The 1919 Nurses' Act developed the supplementary register for "mental nurses" (McGann et al., 31). It was thus "mental nurse" that was prevalent before and during the Second World War nurses and it is the term that will be used predominantly in this essay. Peter Nolan, "Mental Health Nursing – Origins and Developments," in *Nursing and Social Change*, ed. Monica Baly (London: Routledge, 1995); McGann et al., *A History of the Royal College of Nursing*; Nolan & McCrae, *The Story of Nursing in British Mental Hospitals*.

28. Christie, interview by Conrad Wood.

29. Ibid.

30. Claire Chatterton, "'Caught in the Middle'? Mental Nurse Training in England 1919–1951," *Journal of Psychiatric and Mental Health Nursing* 11 (2004): 30–35. It was not only in Britain that the medical profession held power over the mental nurses in a way that it did not over general nursing. The fact that nurses from Dominion countries had similar issues to those in Britain is important given the nature of medical and nursing care provision on active service overseas in the Second World War. For a detailed discussion of gender and professional power disparities psychiatric nursing in Canada in the middle of the 20th century, see Beverley Hicks, "Gender, Politics and Regionalism: Factors in the Evolution of Registered Psychiatric Nursing in Manitoba (1920–1960)," *Nursing History Review, 19* (2011): 103–26.

31. G.M. Robertson, reported from the quarterly meeting of the Medico-Psychological Association on (November 17, 1927) in, "The Status of Mental Nurses," *The Lancet* (December 10, 1927): 1248.

32. Niall McCrae and M. Wright, "Work Rest and Play: Professional and Social Progress of Nurses at a British Mental Hospital in the Early 20th Century," *Journal of Psychiatric and Mental Health Nursing* 23 (2016): 614–23.

33. Neil R. Brimblecombe, "The Changing Relationship between Mental Health Nurses and Psychiatrists in the United Kingdom," *Journal of Advanced Nursing 49*, no. 4 (2005): 344–53.

34. There were exceptions to this. The limited training of nursing sisters in psychiatric care was acknowledged at the time, but their ability to learn quickly brought commendations from the medical staff. Brigadier G.W.B. James, Consultant in Psychological Medicine reported that the sisters were "making an important contribution to the nursing side of psychiatric hospitals … they have always done their duty consistently and well." G.W.B. James, "Extract for Half-Yearly Report, January to (June 1943): Q.A.I.M.N.S. and T.A.N.S. in Psychiatric Nursing," Museum of Military Medicine (MMM) uncatalogued archive.

35. Kylie M. Smith, "Different Places, Different Ideas: Reimagining Practice in American Psychiatric Nursing After World War II," *Nursing History Review 26* (2018): 21.

36. Adams, "The Nursing Role in the Use of Insulin Coma Therapy," 2091.

37. Dingwall et al., *An Introduction to the Social History of Nursing*, 133–34.

38. Chris Hart, *Nurses and Politics: The Impact of Power and Practice* (Basingstoke: Palgrave Macmillan, 2004), 52.

39. Tommy Dickinson, Matt Cook, John Playle & Christine Hallett, "Nurses and Subordination: A Historical Study of Mental Nurses' Perceptions on Administering Aversion Therapy for 'Sexual Deviations,'" *Nursing Inquiry 21*, no. 4 (2013): 287.

40. Penny Summerfield & Corinna Peniston-Bird, "Women in the Firing-Line: The Home Guard and the Defence of Gender Boundaries in Britain in the Second World War," *Women's History Review 9*, no. 2 (2000): 232.

41. Juliette Pattinson, *Behind Enemy Lines: Gender, Passing and the Special Operations Executive in the Second World War* (Manchester: Manchester University Press, 2007),13.

42. Sonya O. Rose, *Which People's War? National Identity and Citizenship in Britain,* (1939–1945) (Oxford: Oxford University Press, 2003).

43. The wearing of trousers by women continued to raise concerns about "mannish" women, fears of moral laxity and the outward sign of women's movement from the domestic environment as men's helpmeet to independence. Deborah Montgomerie, "Assessing Rosie: World War II, New Zealand Women and the Iconography of Femininity," *Gender and History 8*, no. 10 (1996): 118; Lucy Noakes, *Women in the British Army: War and the Gentle Sex* (1907–1948) (London: Routledge, 2006), 116; Martha L. Hall, Belinda T. Orzada, & Dilia Lopez-Gydosh, "American Women's Wartime Dress: Sociocultural Ambiguities Regarding Women's Roles During World War II," *The Journal of American Culture 38*, no. 3 (2015): 237.

44. Betty Crisp interview by Jane Brooks (January 13, 2014), UK Centre for the History of Nursing, University of Manchester (hereafter UKCHN).

45. Gail Braybon and Penny Summerfield, *Out of the Cage: Women's Experiences in Two World Wars* (London: Pandora, 1987), 158.

46. Margaret Parkes, interview by Jane Brooks at her home in the North West of England (December 12, 2012), UKCHN.

47. Penny Summerfield, "Women and War in the Twentieth Century" in, *Women's History: Britain* (1850–1945) ed. June Purvis (London: University College London Press, 1995); Penny Summerfield, *Reconstructing Women's Wartime Lives: Discourse and Subjectivity in Oral Histories of the Second World War* (Manchester: Manchester University Press, 1998).

48. Summerfield, *Reconstructing Women's Wartime Lives*, 88.

49. Pattinson, *Behind Enemy Lines*.

50. Juliette Pattinson, "'Playing the Daft Lassie with Them': Gender, Captivity and the Special Operations Executive During the Second World War," *European Review of History 13*, no. 2 (2006): 276.

51. Joanna Bourke, *The Second World War: A People's History* (Oxford: Oxford University Press, 2001), 1.

52. For full and detailed analysis of the work and growing appreciation of the value of trained nurses in the First World War, see Christine E. Hallett, *Nurse Writers of the Great War* (Manchester: Manchester University Press, 2016); Christine E. Hallett, "'This Fiendish Mode of Warfare': Nursing the Victims of Gas Poisoning in the First World War," in *One Hundred Years of Wartime Nursing Practices* (1954–1953), eds. Jane Brooks & Christine E. Hallett (Manchester: Manchester University Press, 2015); Christine E. Hallett, *Veiled Warriors: Allied Nurses of the First World War* (Oxford: Oxford University Press, 2014); Christine E. Hallett, *Containing Trauma: Nursing Work in the First World War* (Manchester: Manchester University Press, 2009). For a wider review of the work of nursing sisters from Dominion countries, see also, Cynthia Toman, *Sister Soldiers of the Great War: The Nurses*

of the Canadian Army Medical Corps (Vancouver: University of British Columbia Press, 2016); Kirsty Harris, "'Health, Healing and Harmony': Invalid Cookery and Feeding by Australian Nurses in the Middle East in the First World War," in *One Hundred Years of Wartime Nursing Practices* (1954–1953), eds. Jane Brooks & Christine E. Hallett (Manchester: Manchester University Press, 2015); Kirsty Harris, *More than Bombs and Bandages, Australian Army Nurses at Work in World War I* (Newport: Big Sky Publishing, 2011); Ruth Rae, *Scarlet Poppies: The Army Experience of Australian Nurses during World War I* (Burwood: College of Nursing, 2004).

53. John Laffin, *Women in Battle* (London: Abelard Schuman, 1967), 11.

54. Anonymous, "Extract of a Letter to my Wife while Returning from Anzio Beachhead" (March 1944), MMM QARANC uncatalogued archive, CMF file; An officer, "In Step with the QAs. 1.- An Officer Writes to his Wife from the Anzio beachhead," *Nursing Times 40*, 32 (August 5, 1944): 538.

55. Kara Dixon Vuic, "'Officer, Nurse, Woman': Army Nurse Corps Recruitment for the Vietnam War," *Nursing History Review 14* (2006): 135.

56. Noakes, *Women in the British Army*, 126. The exception to this was the use of women in the Special Operations Executive. Although they may have been allotted "female" roles within the SOE, they were in constant danger. Pattinson, *Behind Enemy Lines.*

57. Anonymous nursing sister, "The Anzio Beachhead," MMM QARANC uncatalogued archive, CMF file.

58. Noakes, *Women in the British Army*, 98.

59. Christina Twomey, "Australian Nurse POWs: Gender, War and Captivity," *Australian Historical Studies 36*, no. 124 (2004): 255–274.

60. Jane E. Schultz, *Women at the Front: Hospital Workers in Civil War America* (Chapel Hill: The University of North Carolina Press, 2004), 7.

61. Cynthia Enloe, *Does Khaki Become You? The Militarization of Women's Lives* (London: Pandora, 1988), 213–14.

62. Mary Morris, "The Diary of a Wartime Nurse," (June 19, 1944), 94, IWM Documents.4850; Mary Morris, *A Very Private Diary: A Nurse in Wartime*, ed. Carol Acton (London: Weidenfeld & Nicolson, 2014), 83.

63. Enloe, *Does Khaki Become You?* 106.

64. Sheila M. Bevington, *Nursing Life and Discipline: A Study Based on Over Five Hundred Interviews* (London: H.K. Lewis, 1943), 8.

65. Ann Radloff, "Going to Gooseberry Beach: Travels and Adventures of a Nursing Sister," 1, IWM Documents.147.

66. Brenda McBryde, *A Nurse's War* (Saffron Walden: Cakebread Publications, 1993), 86.

67. Cynthia Enloe argues that military nursing existed on an "ideological knife-edge." Enloe, *Does Khaki Become You?* 106.

68. Joanna Bourke, "Disciplining the Emotions: Fear, Psychiatry and the Second World War," in *War, Medicine and Modernity*, eds. Roger Cooter, Mark Harrison and Steve Sturdy (Stroud: Sutton Publishing, 1998), 225.

69. Crew, "The Army Medical Services," 80.

70. There were no male officer nurses in the Second World War. By the late 1960s, F.A.E. Crew, war historian and later Chair in Social and Preventative Medicine at the University of Edinburgh, argued that he could see this would change: "They [registered male nurses] will certainly seek admission to the Q.A.R.A.N.C. (Queen Alexandra's Royal Army

Nursing Corps) or to the R.A.M.C. (Royal Army Medical Corps) and to find a satisfactory reason for rejecting them will not be at all easy." Crew, "The Army Medical Services," 80.

71. Crew, "The Army Medical Services," 81.

72. Ibid.

73. Marsha L. Burris, *Paradox of Professionalism: American Nurses in World War II* (Charlotte: Spiral Publications, 2007), 96.

74. Hallett, *Containing Trauma*, 158.

75. Ibid, 159.

76. Gilbert Debenham, William Sargant, Denis Hill & Eliot Slater, "Treatment of War Neurosis," *The Lancet* (January 25, 1941): 107.

77. Emma Newlands, *Civilians into Soldiers: War, the Body and British Army Recruits, (1939–1945)* (Manchester: Manchester University Press, 2014), 39. Mark Harrison argues that the idea that certain men were predisposed to mental illness because of their upbringing or hereditary factors was still prevalent at the beginning of the war and some men perpetuated their symptoms of neurosis in order to support claims for discharge on the grounds of ill health with the concomitant pension. Mark Harrison, *Medicine and Victory: British Military Medicine in the Second World War* (Oxford: Oxford University Press, 2004), 59.

78. The debates as to whether men were malingering or not were seen in the nursing press during the early years of the war. In an article for the *Nursing Mirror* in (September 1939), Charles Stanford Read, a physician lecturer in mental illness wrote quite specifically that neurosis should not be associated with malingering: "Suffering on this account is only too real and intense." Charles Stanford Read, "The Nurse and the Psychological Emergencies of War," *Nursing Mirror* (September 16, 1939): 819. In February of the next year, H. Crichton-Miller of the Tavistock Clinic in London, attitude to malingerers was that they valued being ill above being well and then deceived themselves into thinking they were really ill. H. Crichton-Miller, "Psychological Problems of the War as they Affect the Nurse: 2. Neuroses Arising Out of War Conditions," *Nursing Mirror* (17 February 1940): 482–83; Maurice B. Wright, "Psychological Problems of the War as they Affect the Nurse: 3. Conversion Hysteria," *The Nursing Times* (24 February 1940): 510–11.

79. Nell Jarrett, "Diary of her Desert Experiences" (July 25, 1942) (June 21, 1942–January 13, 1943). I am indebted to Nell Jarrett's nephew and niece, Phillip John, his sister Chris and Philip's wife Anna John, for providing me with full access to Sr Jarrett's diary and press cuttings. What is not completely clear is whether Jarrett was only critical of kindly treatment to prisoners of war and whether had they been allied soldiers she would have felt differently.

80. Edgar Jones, "'LMF': The Use of Psychiatric Stigma in the Royal Air Force During the Second World War," *Journal of Military History 70*, no. 2 (2006): 439–58.

81. Harrison, *Medicine and Victory*, 122.

82. Anonymous, "Psychiatric Casualties in Battle," 505–6.

83. Edgar Jones & Simon Wessely, "Psychiatric Battle Casualties: An Intra- and Interwar Comparison," *The British Journal of Psychiatry* 178 (2001): 245.

84. Anonymous, "Nursing in a Psychiatric Hospital for Officers."

85. Edgar Jones & Stephen Ironside, "Battle exhaustion: The Dilemma of Psychiatric Casualties in Normandy (June-August 1944)," *The Historical Journal 53*, no. 1 (2010), p. 109.

86. Notwithstanding this belief, Ben Shephard argues that there was in fact little consensus on who should actually do the selection, "doctors? psychiatrists? officers?" Ben

Shephard, "'Pitiless Psychology': The Role of Prevention in British Military Psychiatry in the Second World War," *History of Psychiatry* x (1999): 505.

87. Newlands, *Civilians into Soldiers: War,* 39.

88. Edgar Jones, "War and the Practice of Psychotherapy: The UK Experience (1939–1960)," *Medical History* 48 (2004): 495.

89. A.H. Ahrenfeldt, "Military Psychiatry," in *Medical Services in War: The Principal Medical Lessons of The Second World War,* eds. Arthur Salusbury MacNalty & W. Franklin Mellor (London: HMSO, 1968), 181.

90. Anonymous, "Psychiatric Casualties in Battle," 505.

91. Jones & Wessely, "Psychiatric Battle Casualties," 243.

92. Kevin Brown, *Fighting Fit: Health, Medicine and War in the Twentieth Century* (Stroud: The History Press, 2008), loc3408. The belief was that the longer the delay in treatment, the poorer the prognosis for the "return to Service duty." Arthur Salusbury MacNalty, "Medicine: Psychological Medicine," in, *Medical Services in War: The Principal Medical Lessons of the Second World War,* eds. Arthur Salusbury MacNalty & W. Franklin Mellor (London: HMSO, 1968), 424.

93. Jones & Wessely, "Psychiatric Battle Casualties," 45; Jones & Ironside, "Battle Exhaustion," 44. Harrison notes that this kindly and perhaps militarily more expedient approach to psychologically damaged men was in stark contrast to the US Army which rapidly returned its psychiatric casualties to battle. Harrison, *Medicine and Victory,* 177.

94. Jones and Ironside argue that a concomitant problem of this, coupled with the limited number of psychiatrists in frontline areas was bed blocking. This led to the transfer of civilian psychiatrists from Britain to military hospitals. Jones & Ironside, "Battle Exhaustion," 116.

95. Jones, "War and the Practice of Psychotherapy," 500.

96. In an article to *Nursing Mirror* in February 1940, Maurice B. Wright told the readers, "First and foremost the patient must not feel that he is thought to be a malingerer." Wright, "Psychological Problems of the War," 510.

97. Catherine Hutchinson, "My War and Welcome to it," 23. IWM Documents.11950.

98. Toman, *An Officer and a Lady,* 152.

99. Morris, "The Diary of a Wartime Nurse" (July 4, 1945), 213; Morris (Acton Ed.) *A Very Private Diary,* 183

100. Stanford Read, "The Nurse and the Psychological Emergencies of War," 319.

101. Ibid, 320.

102. Agnes Kathleen Dunbar Morgan to her Mother (letter 65) (October, 1943), 231, Central Mediterranean Force (CMF), IWM Documents.16686.

103. F.E. Brown to Win & Moll, (August 4, 1944), CMF, IWM Documents.12472

104. Emily Soper, interview by Jane Brooks (September 6, 2013), UKCHN.

105. Morris, "The Diary of a Wartime Nurse" (October 5, 1944), 144; Morris (Acton ed.) *A Very Private Diary,* 127.

106. Soper, interview.

107. Sue Hawkins, *Nursing and Women's Labour in the Nineteenth Century: The Quest for Independence* (London: Routledge, 2010), 22.

108. Evelyn Pearce, *A General Textbook of Nursing: A Comprehensive Guide to the Final State Examinations* (London: Faber & Faber, 1937), 2.

109. James, Extract for Half-Yearly Report, January to June 1943.

110. Sister TANS, "Experiences of an Army Sister in the Middle East: Palestine, Greece, Egypt" (no date), MMM QARANC uncatalogued archive. The TANS were a separate nursing service, having been founded in 1908 as a reserve force. However, during the Second World War they were amalgamated with the Q.A.s. For a more detailed discussion of the founding of the TANS, see Ian Hay, *One Hundred Years of Army Nursing: The Story of the British Army Nursing Services from the Time of Florence Nightingale to the Present Day* (London: Cassell & Company Ltd., 1953), 57.

111. Sister TANS, "Experiences of an Army Sister in the Middle East."

112. One possible reason for the more limited discussions related to the care of psychologically damaged men as opposed to physically damaged ones is the stigma that was attached to mental health and by association those who cared for them. It is likely that the Q.A.s did not wish to be linked to this less distinguished patient group, lest it affect their status too. Claire Chatterton, "'The Weakest Link in the Chain of Nursing'? Recruitment and Retention in Mental Health Nursing in England (1948–1968)," in *Mental Health Nursing: The Working Lives of Paid Carers, 1800s–1900s*, eds. Anne Borsay & Pamela Dale (Manchester: Manchester University Press, 2015), 170.

113. Morgan to her Mother (letter 57) (August, 1943), 4, CMF.

114. In 1949, when senior NCO ex-combatants who had been through extensive war experience, often in the North Africa desert and then into Italy, presented with mental problems, they were labeled as suffering from, "old sergeant syndrome." Jones and Ironside, "Battle Exhaustion," 121.

115. Harrison, *Medicine and Victory*, 172.

116. TANS sister, "Experiences of an Army Sister in the Middle East." The Pioneer Corps was the labor and works corps of the British Army. Their work involved clearing roads, laying tracks, and constructing airfields, roads, and bridges. As well as British recruits, the Pioneer Corps comprised men from the then British colonies as well as German and Austrian Jews who had fled Nazi Europe.

117. TANS sister, "Experiences of an Army Sister in the Middle East."

118. Morris, "The Diary of a Wartime Nurse," June 28, 1944, 116; Morris, (Acton ed.) *A Very Private Diary*, 100.

119. Morris, "The Diary of a Wartime Nurse," June 28 and June 26, 1944, 113; Morris (Acton ed.), *A Very Private Diary*, 99 & 96.

120. Morris, "The Diary of a Wartime Nurse," January 27, 1945, 170; Morris (Acton ed.), *A Very Private Diary*, 147.

121. Morris, "The Diary of a Wartime Nurse," June 24, 1944, 110; Morris (Acton ed.), *A Very Private Diary*, 95.

122. Anonymous, "Where Minds Are Cured," *Nursing Times* (October 2, 1943): 738–39.

123. Unlike Occupational therapy, active rehabilitation through physiotherapy was a relatively new concept. Physiotherapy may have grown out of massage at the beginning of the 20th century, but the idea of it as an active treatment, that could return men to work or war, expanded the horizons of its practitioners. Julie Anderson, *War, Disability and Rehabilitation in Britain: 'Soul of a Nation'* (Manchester: Manchester University Press, 2011).

124. Patricia D'Antonio, "Relationships, Reality and Reciprocity with Therapeutic Environments: A Historical Case Study," *Archives of Psychiatric Nursing* XVIII, no. 1 (2004): 11–16.

125. Harris, *More than Bombs and Bandages,* loc4078; Linker, *War's Waste,* 71; Ana Carden-Coyne, *The Politics of Wounds: Military Patients and Medical Power in the First World War* (Oxford: Oxford University Press, 2014), 264–69.

126. British Red Cross Society and the Order of St. John of Jerusalem, *War Organisation: Third Annual Report,* (1941–1942)*, Together with The Report of the Finance Sub-Committee and the Statement of Accounts and the Third Annual Report of The Duke of Gloucester's Red Cross and St John Fund and the Accounts of the Fund* (London: British Red Cross Society and Order of Sister John of Jerusalem, 1943), 15.

127. Carden-Coyne, *The Politics of Wounds,* 269.

128. Anderson, *War, Disability and Rehabilitation in Britain,* 78.

129. I.B.H., "In Step with the Q.A.s. 2.," 557.

130. Ibid.

131. Elsie Driver to Miss Soutar, July 9, 1944, MMM QARANC uncatalogued archive.

132. Toman, *An Officer and a Lady,* 152.

133. Anonymous, "Where Minds Are Cured," 739.

134. R.D. Gillespie, "A Critical Review: Narcosis Therapy," *Journal of Neurology, Neurosurgery & Psychiatry 2* (1939): 47.

135. According to Harrison, by 1943 specialist psychiatric nurses were posted to the Western desert, a date that approximates with Driver's posting to the desert. It may be that Harrison is correct, but the psychiatrically trained nursing sisters were not made available to Driver's hospital. However, this is not clear from the limited evidence available.

136. Driver to Soutar, (July 9, 1944).

137. Ibid.

138. Angus MacNiven, "The Nursing of Mental Illness," in *War-Time Nurse: An Anthology of Ideas about the Care and Nursing of War Casualties,* ed. J.M. Mackintosh (Edinburgh: Oliver & Boyd, 1940), 161.

139. Nolan & McCrae, *The Story of Nursing in British Mental Hospitals,* 102.

140. I.B.H., "In Step with the Q.A.s. 2," 557.

141. Pentothal was a particularly dangerous treatment as its accumulative effect could lead to death. However, when this became fully appreciated is not known. In late 1943 and early 1944, one of Sister Catherine Hutchinson's patients was given IV pentothal as an anaesthetic for severe pain: "Which unknown to the MOs had a cumulative action. After several days he died, mostly from the build up of anaesthetic. The medical staff were shattered, but at least had learnt a valuable lesson about the dangers of powerful drugs." Hutchinson, "My War and Welcome to it."

142. Gillespie, "A Critical Review: Narcosis Therapy," 47.

143. I.B.H., "In Step with the Q.A.s. 2," 557.

144. TANS sister, "Experiences of an Army Sister in the Middle East."

145. I.B.H., "In Step with the Q.A.s. 2," 557. According to Jesper Vaczy Kragh, Danish psychiatrists started to use hypertherm in 1942, but it never replaced malarial therapy as the electricity necessary made it too expensive. Jesper Vaczy Kragh, "Malaria Fever Therapy for General Paralysis of the Insane in Denmark," *History of Psychiatry 21,* no. 4 (2010): 480. Malarial treatment for general paralysis of the insane, or neurosyphilis was used form the 1920s to the 1950s. The purpose of the treatment was to create a hyperpyrexia to kill the syphilis spirochete and stop the disease process. However, even in its early days, there were concerns about the ethics of such treatment. Mathew Gambino suggests

that even as early as 1930, some physicians were equivocal regarding the use of malarial therapy and research into its efficacy: Matthew Gambino, "Fevered Decisions: Race, Ethics, and Clinical Vulnerability in the Malarial Treatment of Neurosyphilis (1922–1953)," *Hastings Center Report* 45, no. 4 (2015): 44.

146. Harrison argues that in North Africa and the Central Mediterranean Force (CMF), sedation, including narcosis therapy had become, "a major part of the psychiatrists' repertoire." Harrison, *Medicine and Victory*, 178.

147. Anonymous, "Psychiatric Casualties in Battle," 505.

148. Noakes, *Women in the British Army*, 7. See also John Laffin, "Epilogue," *Women in Battle*, 184–85.

149. Morgan to her Mother (letter 50), "Obeying our General's Orders"; Brenda McBryde, *Quiet Heroines: Nurses of the Second World War* (London: Chatto & Windus, 1985), 126.

150. In Crew's "The Army Medical Services," there are a range of quotations from medical military men on both the problems and the value of having female nurses in forward areas. Crew, "The Army Medical Services," 77–81.

151. Anonymous, "Topical Notes—Normandy Broadcast," *The Nursing Times* (July 1, 1944): 430.

JANE BROOKS
Senior Lecturer
The University of Manchester
Oxford Rd
Manchester
M13 9PL

Cold Interests, Hot Conflicts: How a Professional Association Responded to a Change in Political Regimes

RICARDO A. AYALA
Ghent University

MARKUS THULIN
University of Cologne

E. ROCÍO NÚÑEZ
University of Santiago de Chile

Abstract. In South America, the 1970s began with ardent sociopolitical crises leading to a wave of repressive military regimes. In Chile, most professional bodies suffered profound structural and functional modifications resulting from internal political polarization as well as state intervention. Nurses saw the same fate befall them, which created both a historical blackout and abrupt changes in power dynamics. Given the prominence of this process in the reconfiguration of modern nursing's identity, this article traces the association's political process during the short-lived 1970s Marxist-inspired government and the response of nurses collectively to the rapid shift into a repressive regime leading to a profound internal crisis and an identity break-up within nursing. By using archival sources and oral testimonies[1] of 1970s and 1980s nurses, we reconstruct a historical account of a key period in the history of the country that for the nurses meant a progression of discord and division along with a self-imposed silence on the past. In so doing, the article adds to a growing literature on the participation of women in political life.

The 1970s and 1980s were one of the most turbulent periods in the history of contemporary nursing in Chile.[2] After enjoying an era of steady formal-

Nursing History Review 27 (2019): 57–86. A Publication of the American Association for the History of Nursing. Copyright © 2019 Springer Publishing Company.
http://dx.doi.org/10.1891/1062-8061.27.57

ization, recognition and growth since the early 20th century, the national scenario of regime switch altered the institutionality of the profession, leading to internal political polarization and, eventually, to an unexpected break-up.[34] A national project of Marxist-inspired centralization of welfare services and redistribution of wealth and power in 1970 escalated rapidly to a peak of civil upheaval and subsequent military intervention in 1973, with the President (Salvadore Allende) being overthrown in a *coup d'état*, and the Commander-in-Chief of the Military (Augusto Pinochet) coming to power as the Head of State by declaring a state of siege.

Part of the immediate measures involved political repression, including the suppression of the National Parliament, the outlawing of all political parties, and forceful control over public services, universities, and other professional bodies. Although most professional associations had denounced the economical and social consequences of the former socialist regime and were supportive toward the restoration of public order, they also suffered military intervention in their functioning. Nurses were no exception, and this development meant both internal political polarization and a self-imposed silence on history and memory.[5]

As was the case elsewhere, many of the elements of change contained in this history were part of a global shift in power. This article reconstructs the political reconfiguration of the nursing profession in Chile, focusing on the 1970–1986 timespan. The focus upon these decades intends to unravel nurses' response to regime switches, flows of power, alliances, social movements, decision-making, influences, and relations within the State. Whereas it is often assumed that women had a passive, apolitical positioning during this period of extreme political transformation,[6] this article gives an example of women's active participation in the public sphere.

In reconstructing this political history, we draw, on the one hand, upon testimonies of nurses from the 1970s and 1980s exploring experiences, relations, and responses in our period of interest; and on the other hand on documents retrieved through manual searches of the archives of the Chilean Nursing Association (*Colegio de Enfermeras de Chile*), and extensive searches in external sources such as the National Library of Chile, the Library of the Ministry of Health, and the Library of the National Congress, comprising press clippings, photographs, public statements, letters, and classified cables, among other documents.

The article is structured as follows: after providing the details of our methodological approach, we present the findings of a study exploring the main five political developments that nurses underwent in just a two-decade span, namely: (a) relatively stable ambience of political heterogeneity in the frame of increasingly statist public policies; (b) the position of the professional association toward the Marxist-inspired regime; (c) the Nurses Association's loss of control over the nurses during the military regime; (d) the process of resistance exerted by groups of nurses; and (e) a challenging scenario of negotiations with the military. Through these areas, we highlight the challenges that—as women—nurses faced and the strategies that allowed them to endure and overcome the political crisis. While the article adds a novel contribution to the understanding of modern nursing in Chile, it also contributes to a growing body of literature that utterly reverses stories and common assumptions about women as apolitical individuals.

The Sources: A Note on Methodology

This study was concerned with the reconfiguration of flows of power, among nurses, between opposing groups of nurses, and between the nurses association and the state. Therefore, our approach was twofold. First, we gathered archives that were extrinsic to nursing with which to build a contextual framework for the recent past; in so doing, we did manual searches in the archive section of the Chilean National Library, and digitized archive collections retrieved from the same library, the Library of Congress of Chile, the Library of the Ministry of Health, and digitized newspaper and magazine collections. We also consulted the archives of international organizations, such as the Red Cross, the Pan American Health Organisation, the International Council of Nurses, and foreign universities. And second, we included narratives from a standpoint intrinsic to nursing by using interviews with a group of nurses who worked through the 1970s and 1980s. After obtaining approval from the respective ethics committee, the interviewees were given a description of the study and, after consenting, a timeline to register facts and landmarks they considered important for changes in power.

The analysis was based on four dimensions: orientation, complication, evaluation, result and ending. Ours was an interpretive political history oriented not only by historical–biographical approaches,[7] but also by a feminist political history approach[8] more broadly, as we focused purposively on the narratives of professional women, largely excluded from narratives of political processes.

The combination of methods expanded our understanding of the problem. While compiling archives enables a reconstruction of facts, actors and sequence of events, testimonies show how historical circumstances shape people's "world in common" with reference to the facts.[9] This strategy helped us overcome the limitations of using a single source and interpret historically produced realities more accurately.

Relatively Stable Ambience of Politically Heterogeneous Ideas

For much of the 20th century, the nursing profession as we know it today grew steadily and strengthened as welfare services became consolidated. Social policies beginning in the late 1920s and the creation of the National Health Service (NHS) in the mid-1950s offered the setting in which nurses fought poverty and insalubrity in the community and ran the wards in hospitals. Whereas in the 1860s, the Chilean population was overwhelmingly rural, by the 1960s about 70% of Chileans lived in urban areas, a move that accentuated problems of public sanitation and living conditions.[10] This increased nurses' awareness of their social mandate, while public health nursing gained salience through health reforms endorsed by a number of medical doctors trained in Europe. Nurses would then take part in the "social mothership" of well-to-do ladies.[3]

Nurses were regarded in a positive light and, in fact, enjoyed the backing of Liberal and Christian Democrat governments alike, while being considered a necessary but scarce resource. A number of landmarks were achieved in this period. For example, the creation of the Chilean Nurses Association in 1953—meant to decouple a former trade union with other practitioners—the increase from 45 to 80 in the capacity of new students at the NHS School of Nursing[11] and permission for specializations granted in 1965[12] thanks to funding from the United States,[13] a policy that was complemented with the strengthening of the training for Red Cross nurses, the organization of hospital volunteer work by ladies (i.e. *Damas de Rojo*), and the increase of hospital beds available throughout the country.

Up until 1970, there was continuity in dominant sociopolitical ideas in the national scene, which would only be interrupted for 6 years in 1958 by a right-wing government that implemented austerity measures affecting, among other aspects, the wages of public employees. And yet the nursing profession seemed to be the perfect match for the big scheme of public policy ideologically. Both Christian humanist and nationalist values dominated Chilean politics, with the nursing profession—along with social workers—engraining fully in that setting and consolidating its selfless identity and its commitment toward the social fabric. The interest of some nurses in political life is very telling in this respect. In 1941, Gladys Peake—who would become very influential in the affairs of a number of nursing initiatives as well as in the health bureaucracy—was a candidate for the post of Representative of the Valparaiso District on a Socialist ticket[14][15] (although soon after this was used against her when applying to the Rockefeller Foundation—which was capitalist in nature—depicting her as "too political" and therefore inappropriate as a potential fellow).[16] Other nursing leaders endorsed similar ideologies; for example, by participating in women's movements, such as the Chilean Feminine Party, one of the groups backing the campaign of President Ibáñez del Campo, elected in 1952, which would pave the way for the creation of the Chilean Nurses Association in the year to come. Nurse Rosalba Flores also had ties to the broader movement for the women's right to vote,[17] which proposed a law that was passed in 1949. These movements were also closely linked to a number of other female groups that gathered pharmacists, midwives, social workers, and physiotherapists, and facilitated the strengthening of their professional associations in the same period.

By coming into contact with key national leaders such as Elena Pedraza and Ana Figueroa, nurses took their first steps into political partaking. Indeed, an important milestone was their participation in the 1950 national strike,[18] the single most important one of the era, which not only fed fears of destabilization among politicians but also aligned workers with left-wing ideals.[19] However, nurses did not consider themselves as blue-collar workers and only occasionally engaged in strikes and public demonstrations in this period. For, in fact, their status as a graduate profession prompted the formal detachment from the non-university-trained health workforce in a time when access to higher education was highly selective.

In the next decade, the leadership of the Chilean Nurses Association maintained a center–right position, with a sympathizer of the Christian Democratic Party, Marilia Fonseca, chairing the Board for two consecutive terms. Toward the end of her second term, Silvia Alessandri, a National Party candidate in 1967 Santiago elections for Representatives and niece of a former rightist President, handled the women's vote, topping the list of 81 candidates. She had a strong affinity with women's associations and the healthcare sector, as she was herself a Red Cross nurse. This, too, may have induced some identification with conservative ideas within the Nurses Association. Interestingly, the far left never actually had the chance to weigh in on the Association's affairs. Either because their voice was silenced for not fitting the national value frame—the Communist Party had even been formally banned in the country for 10 years—or because nurses felt that their necessities did not echo the realities of industrial workers.

Nevertheless, as public services gained more prominence and nurses became a key resource in public health,[20] this assortment of political views in the Association reflects a rather harmonious relation between nurses and the state, and among nurses themselves. Conflict, if any existed, did not transpire into the public sphere, and in fact did not restrain the flourishing of the profession in this era. Nurses managed to install their agendas in different instances, as Board members were often faculty nurses, ministry advisors, members of supranational health entities, and visiting fellows in US and Canadian universities. Their strategic presence would garner sufficient legislative support across governments and bolster self-regulation.

Change of Winds: A Marxist-Inspired Regime

On the eve of 1970 elections, the main heading of the Illustrated Daily News read, "All Chile will give him absolute majority," as a picture of conservative candidate Arturo Alessandri waving the hordes dominated the cover.[21] On the other side, leaflets distributed by supporters of the leftist conglomerate *Unidad Popular* (UP) publicized, "Let's raise people's power," along with images of raised fists, and the sickle and hammer sign. As uncommon as it appeared, Chile was in the spotlight, and international observers followed the news minutely—if Allende was to win the elections, this would be the first Marxist government ever coming to power through democratic voting. Trade unions were hopeful. But nurses, not necessarily so.

Nurses knew that their most enthusiastic supporters, those who made their professional association possible,[22] were mostly connected to the center–right. The professions, it was perceived, were an important part of the economy, and, in fact, the late 1940s and early 1950s became the era of "the associative movement in Chile,"[23] leading to a number of newly created professional associations. Whereas the social reforms initiated in the 1920s represented a combination of principles of social hygiene and ideals of social welfare, the nation was now between two opposing ideologies: the one encouraging structural modifications for a more liberal economy under the patronage of the US government, and the other inciting a proletarian revolution inspired by the Soviet Union and Cuba. The Communist Party in Chile had grown to be the subcontinent's largest in proportion to population.[24]

The future role and status of nurses in either scenario was rather unclear, mostly because they were caught in a sociopolitical limbo, not fully recognized at the level of other health professions but not self-ascribed as laborers either. Along with pharmacists, biochemists, and dentists, in 1962 the Chilean Medical Association had been conferred a special legal status (see Act 15.076) that, aside from securing medical care, legitimized higher wages, and attractive career benefits. This development reinforced a sense of status elevation on the part of nurses, who struggled to obtain the same functionary status in the state bureaucracy, without succeeding in the negotiations throughout two different governments. Nevertheless, if bargaining ways to the Chamber was to be continued, having UP lawmakers paying attention to nurses' claims would mean an uphill battle. Not least, because the left wing was the main detractor of women's right to voting, since the female movement was often identified with conservative ideas. Indeed, it was elite right-wing women who engaged in politics most often, as they could afford the necessary time and resources.[25] In an interview with researcher I. Berliner,[26] a former nursing lead recalls:

> I can still remember the terror-spreading campaign for women not to vote for Allende in 1970, even though I didn't want to vote for him. I knew him as a Senator, a very smart and pleasant person, somebody who did a lot for healthcare, the pregnant women, the consumptive patients, etc.[27]

Although in the past nurses had been lobbying with a young Allende as the Minister of Sanitation,[28] the attempts of the now older presidential candidate to adopt a socialist order did not seem to be the best case scenario. For, in fact, the socialist project was regarded with disdain by most professional associations, as socialism itself gained more militants and sympathizers among the youths (i.e. the Communist Youth of Chile) and the marginalized (i.e. the Farmers' Union). Professional groups feared that the rise of Marxist structuralism could raise the issue of the position of the professions in the division of labor as an extension of the hierarchy of social classes. Hence, the professional associations became one of the most important interest groups in an environment of increasing polarization of worldviews throughout a decade. Internally, associations' boards were often configured using party politics as a blueprint and the elections patterns often reflected national trends. Therefore, ideas within nursing were likely to have, too, shifted gradually leftwards, but without being able to work their way through the Association's National Board.

The leftward trend regained prominence from 1964 through 1970, with candidates achieving 23.3% of votes in the parliamentary elections of 1965, the highest in six consecutive elections. With the right wing attracting the lowest figures in over three decades, this political landscape could only be the prelude for another result to come 5 years later: the victory of Salvador Allende as the Head of State.

Nurses Lose Control over the Association

Public life during the UP period was characterized by a perceptible tense atmosphere, given the difficulties of the government to control soaring inflation, the economic speculation circulated by the opposition, and the external interventionism in national politics. These were orchestrated by state policies of nationalization of industries and a Church-promoted program of expropriation and redistribution of land.

In the public debate, detractors accused a proposed plan for a totally integrated education system along with the nationalization of the paper-making industry would establish a Marxist doctrinaire monopoly, whereas UP supporters argued that supplies of the food market were blocked by the conservatives who lived on their own hidden stock, as part of their manoeuvres to block the presidency. Meanwhile, the *New York Times* fanned the fear machine by announcing to the world, "Chile restores formal ties with Cuba; End of alignment with U.S. policy seen."[29] On both sides, discourse had a pessimistic undertone of urgency.

And the situation on a day-to-day level was indeed urgent. General strikes, marches and factory occupations were organized every so often, with the resulting intervention from the police, as housewives—or maids on their behalf—had to queue endlessly for food and groceries in the midst of the acute supply crisis. According to the national press, all professional associations went on strike to protest, and nurses' oral testimonies lead us to the view that most nurses participated in the national strikes of October 1972 and August 1973—the whole healthcare sector was mobilized by the Medical Association (*Colegio Médico*). Nevertheless, some nurses remained loyal to the government, either joining UP political campaigns or not following the calls for strikes against the Allende administration. Across classes and parties, it was felt that as a former Ministry of Health, Allende understood the scarcity of a professional nursing workforce.[30] In fact, over 300 study opportunities were offered as evening programs for health workers in 1972, among which 125 were devoted to nursing.[31,32]

However, as a right-wing Board took office at the Chilean Nurses Association in 1971, lobbying activities to acquire a higher legal status for the profession intensified. Claims were made before the Parliament by Christian Democrat Senator Ricardo Valenzuela Sáez on August 28, 1973[33] and then again on September 6 of the same year[34] at the request of the Association. The aim was to circumscribe the scope of nurses' professional practice and establish penalties for usurpation. This was no superfluous move, for it surfaced[35] that in the middle of a convoluted ambience of protests and strikes against the sociopolitical crisis,[36] the Association's justification for joining the strikes was rather peculiar, given the larger picture: that of being included in an umbrella law for health professionals, instead of remaining with nonuniversity workers in the same regulation. Being perceived in a parallel relation with medical doctors was thus important, and the social turmoil offered a setting for less attention-catching strategies. They operated behind the scenes and did not often engage in broader public debates.

But the Association's efforts proved tiresome and ineffective. The Board members grew increasingly discontented with the regime, which augmented their anti-UP stance and not only strengthened their ties with a larger confederation of 19 professional associations (CUPROCH)[37] but also refreshed relations with movements of rightist women,[38][39] both seeking to overthrow the UP leader. Along with industry-owners, the professional associations became a chief middle-class social force in the public sphere in the 1972–1973 period,[40] with nursing among the rare female groups.

The defeat of the UP government is too well known to deserve much attention here.[41] What is important to highlight, however, is that CUPROCH acknowledged[42] that their movement accentuated the tensions that led to the overthrow of Allende on September 11, 1973. Radical on many levels, there is a sense in which the changes of regimes of the 1970s mirrored international politics of the Cold War. The nurses' status issue thus added to the perception of the, now defeated, UP as a "godless" anti-private property force.

Unsurprisingly then, the switch into a liberal economy under a repressive regime seemed to promise a new chance for nurses to realize their aspirations. Key in this process was a fiercely anti-socialist nursing lead: General Secretary Gladys Peake. She had radically changed her worldviews during her stay in the United States, and now appeared repeatedly lobbying with politicians to have the Association's voice heard at the National Parliament and controlling the communications with nurses across the country. Equally, she was responsible for hiring the nursing staff onto the NHS: "I was surprised she was in her advanced age when she interviewed me at the NHS, but still so very active and meticulous."[43] By examining the archives closely, one gains the impression that she was a "de facto president" who controlled the doings of the Association and that all the important decisions had to be consented by her. Peake's political involvement went as far as to serve as one of the handpicked delegates before the International Labour Organization during the Pinochet administration[44][45] and to have formal bonds with a conservative sector that sought to forge a renovated right wing (*Movimiento de Unión Nacional*).[46]

Written soon after the *coup d'état*, three documents seem to be of crucial importance in understanding the significant rightwards shift of the Nurses Association's board. First, President Sonia Garrido Ballerino signed in December 1973, together with other rightist female professional leads, a public statement acknowledging the military for liberating the nation from Marxism and the "consequent permanent climate of disorder, violence and terrorism."[47] Second, and in the same trimester, the Chilean Nurses Association published its first statement about the *coup* in its *Boletín Informativo*, including a flattering letter[48] sent to the very Augusto Pinochet, the new Head of State, signed by Sonia Garrido and Gladys Peake on December 7. In the letter they raised again their concern about the legal frame for the profession; they complained that the former government did not make any decision on the issue and that negotiations on a law project were interrupted by the military involvement "that saved our fatherland from the Marxist dictatorship." On the same page, a succinct answer from Pinochet signed a fortnight later is included,[49] where he stated that the salaries of nurses would be analysed in light of the [unhealthy] economic situation of the country. Clearly, he furnished no consideration for the law nurses sought.

Noticeably, when addressing nursing fellows, the *Boletín* Editor-in-Chief, Rosalba Flores, speaks of a "national reconstruction"[50]—a term coined by the Military Junta;[51] her word choice indicates the ideological alignment of the Board with the government. Likewise, the same magazine includes the response of the President of the Association, Sonia Garrido, to a letter of the Nicaraguan Nurses Association—also under a repressive regime—explaining there was "false information [accusations against the Military] being spread by certain individuals and organs of the foreign press." She also wrote to the United Nations defending what she considered to be "the truth"[52] behind the charges. Nationwide, exchanges also continued, as shown by the close contact between Gladys Peake, in her role as the Chief-representative of the nurses at the NHS, with Lidia Díaz, Chief-representative of the nurses at the Pan American Health Organization.[53][54]

While these representatives run political maneuvers, their correspondence shows they knew exactly who to address both nationally and internationally.

Moreover, they knew about the accusations of violations of human rights in Chile circulated by the international press and were quick to claim those were false. The need for commitment toward the military government was evident since their political latitude had proved insufficient in the past. They tightened their internal measures by offering the government longer working hours on behalf of all nurses across the country—although no consultation was made by the Board—for the sake of "national reconstruction,"[55] as one of our interviewees cried, albeit blaming the administration:

> So … then all that happened in 1973, our working ours went up, from just 6 hours the health service increased them to 8 hours per day.[56]

This added to the contribution of the nursing profession. In a sense, the military always had the need to appoint high-ranking nurses (often relatives of Generals of the army) to the Ministry of Health,[57] possibly in an attempt to keep stability within the system as reforms began to be planned. That was the case at least until the early 1980s. Another interviewee explained how easy it was for the leaders to simply tell nurses what had been decided:

> We [some practice nurses] weren't … weren't really interested in syndicalism and the like; that was wrong perhaps, because we weren't committed to what the leaders were doing, so we just did as told [by them].[58]

And third, in a report about the 1977 Congress of the International Council of Nurses held in Tokyo, the then President of the Chilean Nurses Association, Viviana Corrales, was reported to be particularly supportive toward the military regime, "giving the impression that she was there to speak highly of the government, and evading its fundamental political problem," and that Corrales "distributed political propaganda at the end of the congress."[59] Her participation was not well looked upon, especially by commentator M. Eugenia Somalo, a Spanish co-attendee who considered that Corrales avoided the fundamental problem in her country despite being "much criticized all over the world." According to Somalo, she went as far as evading the ICN proposal of integrating the nursing profession into the political situation of each country. Worth noting is that 2 years earlier Tokyo had hosted the 29th General Assembly of the World Medical Association, whose core theme on medical torture was very much present in the global agenda. Somalo also condemned Corrales for filling up her presentation with off-topic technical information about Chilean nursing and failing to engage with the ICN's purpose.

Despite this entire agenda, the situation would only become worse in the years to come, as the authority—and thus the right to grant licence to practice—of all professional associations was suppressed by the government.[60] They could no longer supervise their members—by this token the government sought to discourage unionism.

Thus far, the analysis brings the following two insights in regard to the intertwinement between nurses' aspirations and the political developments of the time. On the one hand, the Board members actively operated as an interest group at different levels to have the attention of legislators during different governments and *across* different political leanings. And on the other hand, as the results demonstrated, nurses' tactics regarding major legal changes were unfruitful irrespective of those political leanings. However, appropriate or inappropriate their political involvement may seem, this development demonstrates the dynamic political action of nurses as an important part of the educated female workforce.

Social Movements of Nurses under the Repressive Regime: Power and Resistance

Having shed light on nurses' devices to wield power, it is necessary to discuss another concomitant political process during the repressive regime: that of resistance. When the Military Junta took office, on September 11, 1973, one of its first measures was to enforce a strict curfew and forbid political gatherings and all activities in public places that could incite disturbances, including universities, hospitals, and other nursing workplaces. One of our interviewees recalls: "It was so frightening, most of us just worked with our heads bowed in bitterness as some friends and comrades were disappearing. We had to be extremely careful what to tell… and to whom."[61] Figures give a clear picture of the social atmosphere: over 3,000 people were brought to military courts or sentenced to prison, and over 2,000 were murdered.[62] Torture was a common measure of the rulers to track their political adversaries, nearly half of them congregated in the Socialist Party, the Communist Party, and the Movement of the Revolutionary Left (MIR). A moral value problem was evident in the national spirit.

Against this background, it was unusual that in March 1974 the first post-*coup* issue of the Nursing Association's trade magazine, *Revista Enfermería*, circulated the text of an international oath for nurses to be used in graduation ceremonies. Similarly, in this usually nonpolitical medium, Editor-in-Chief,

Gladys Peake, requested nurses' commitment to take care of every person "without distinction of race, religion, political position or social condition."[63] While the publication of this piece may seem strange, it is likely a response to reminders from international humanitarian organizations to respect human dignity, organizations such as the International Committee of the Red Cross[64] and Amnesty International.[65] Given the international reach of cases of human rights violations in Chile, executives at the International Council of Nurses formalized their position in written form in 1975.[66] At all levels, including the Presidency and the Military Court, official discourses were that human rights were being protected. The Board of the Nurses Association may have been aware of human rights violations by medical personnel, the same that they had denied in earlier letters. And yet the nature of this information was too delicate to be registered. International observers were also concerned about the detention, persecution, and torture of medical personnel themselves—those who had not sabotaged Allende's plans in hospitals became a common target of the Military.

Whereas the early post-*coup* time might appear as an orderly era when nurses had no participation other than increasing their weekly working hours, they were still very active in political life. The Nurses Association announced in December 1973 the creation of appeals committees at the regional divisions (*Comisiones de Apelación de los Consejos Regionales*) aimed at detecting cases in which fellow nurses may have lost their jobs or been brought to prison without any antecedent of "direct political activity." The goal of those committees was to impede "punishments other than a transfer to another unit." In the context of a dictatorship where a large portion of society participated, ruling groups' calls for humanity and neutrality are believed to be a mere façade. However, this reflects the atmosphere of fear and repression, especially in the first year of the military rule, which also focused on some nurses' antecedents and the eventual resistance they would be able to exert.

Police and military raids often included torture and forced disappearances, but this was steadily denied by the authorities and systematically omitted in the official media, which was the usual attitude throughout the regime. Active resistance, however, was exerted by a number of individual nurses. That was the case of Communist nurse Hilda Velásquez, murdered together with her family in September 1973.[67] The same fate would befall Socialist nurse Waldo Alfaro, rumoured to keep an arsenal of medical instruments in his house and murdered in 1974, and four nursing students.[68]

A number of other nurses[69] were arrested, interrogated and occasionally persecuted, threatened with death, harassed, judged, exiled, tortured, or subjected to vexation. In other cases, they were simply barred from being hired onto the public system.[70] The Board members chose collaboration with the Military and, in many ways, failed to protect all of the nurses. Here, an internal opposition group would become very influential toward the mid-1980s—the Santiago Region branch of the Nurses Association—which actively advocated for the affected nurses while joining an interprofessional union called the *Asamblea de la Civilidad*. In an interview with the National Museum of Memory and Human Rights, its then leaders explained their clandestine work in convincing other nurses and creating bonds with resisting groups from other professional associations and wider social movements despite the "witch hunt"[71] that characterized the resistance period. For example, two activist nurses, G. Corral and M. Reusch, were arrested in 1986 on the grounds of spreading "false accusations of murder against the police"[72,73] (the *degollados* case), condemning afterwards the National Board for "celebrating" the fact in their trade magazine. Worth is noting that the Board members had warned nurses in 1973 that they would not intervene when sanctions were applied by the authorities "in cases of noticeable public political activism";[74] that is, left-wing activism. Acknowledging the Military and pressuring nurses to take a stance, their stance, would set the tone for making up one "official" voice, their voice, for nurses in the public sphere. Interviewees working at the time in different areas of practice recall:

> There was a black hand operating at the university, and in fact I severely criticised that this university didn't protect its academics from the Military measures … and in other places that was even worse, some professors would be just taken out and never be seen again.[75]
>
> At the community health centers, we were impeded from doing our activities, because they suspected we, nurses, could be able to do activism with the people, and so on. Home visits were then forbidden.[76]

This control model was then extended to the regional divisions, although the power was disproportionally concentrated in the National Board. Likewise, contrary to the 1981 Act on professional associations that allowed autonomous internal elections, subsequent Presidents Carmen Oye, Sonia Garrido and Elizabeth Gudelhoeffer (as well as the 10-year General Secretary Gladys Peake) consistently refused legal representation of any nurse involved in a movement that was critical to the government.[77]

Ironically though, the strict curfew, which lasted over 13 years, brought resisting activists together. Behind closed doors, they could more safely discuss their ideas and plan their strategies during clandestine gatherings. Similarly, Andean music was typically a medium to feed, spread and represent resistance against the dictatorship, which was facilitated by a Moscow-controlled radio station that aired Marxist talk shows and news. These were important mechanisms that our interviewees recall, through which they accessed resisting groups and learnt from them.

Looking at the situation with this background in mind, it is easier to understand how fractured the Chilean Nurses Association was—the Board members, on the one hand, acting dutifully to assist those who were believed to have saved the nation and supported market freedom, and resisting nurses, on the other hand, struggling to organize clandestinely since they thought of that as the way back to democracy. While other views somewhere in between were voiced,[78] these two were the main political forces striving to reach balance within the Association.

Negotiations in the Wake of the Healthcare Reforms of 1978–1982 and End of an Era

With the Military in power, there came an inevitable structural reform of the State. Reforms not only have organizational effects; they also bring to the fore interests and values, and the strategies with which to protect them. Despite early significant cuts to public spending for the healthcare system, structural changes did not occur until 1978. Contemporary author Llambias-Wolff illuminated these matters by arguing that lobby groups in the Medical Association and the Air Force exerted overwhelming control over social policy, and in the process extended the status quo.[79]

From 1978 through 1982, the Military Junta implemented a profound transformation of social welfare sectors, especially in healthcare, education, and the pension system.[80] During 1979 and 1980, the then centralized NHS was replaced by a conglomerate of decentralized region-based divisions—the National System of Health Services—while the public health insurance was organized in a separate central entity.[81] Both these arrangements operated autonomously under the supervision of the Ministry of Health. In 1981, the legal scaffolding for a new system of private insurance companies was set. In the same year, the administration of primary care centers became a responsibility of the 341 municipalities throughout the country.

An additional significant move was the change in the financing mechanisms of public sector providers. From 1978 to 1981, a payment-per-delivered-service system was introduced, and hospitals and municipalities were reimbursed retrospectively based on a list of prices for medical interventions and primary care procedures.[82] But this system, again, neglected nurses' prerogatives. Anticipating the results, Gladys Peake, Alicia Cartes Aguilera, Sofía Matus Lagos, and Lidia Díaz undertook a major study on the nursing workforce in 1979, for want of a better way to improve the conditions of nursing careers.[83] Their data ranged from 1974 onwards and gave an overview of nursing work in hospitals and rural centers in the areas of Rancagua, Talca, and Valparaíso. Unsurprisingly, they demonstrated serious shortages of nurses in all areas; even on the secondary and tertiary levels, nursing care could not be guaranteed. It is unknown whether this study was read by the Military, but it is believed that it most surely was. However, the dramatic situation of care services was ignored and the health workforce was progressively reduced throughout the 1980s, in the frame of the most drastic reform of the sector since 1952.[84]

By 1990, the proportion of private healthcare grew up to 25%. Only about 10% of the insured were covered by other public agencies (Army Health Service, university health services, etc.), with the majority of the population receiving medical care from the State-run system. Therefore, most nurses were still employed in the public sector, although affected collectively by challenging conditions in three main areas—political representation, wages, and academic training. These areas affected nurses.

First, the Military selected, controlled closely and scrutinized the personal lives of the nursing staff, which was aggravated by stripping the professional associations of their status as part of the state bureaucracy while taking away most of their attributions. This meant that associations would no longer have actual control over their members. The ending of the once powerful NHS also meant the suppression of an integrated nursing service, and thus the direct defence of the interests of the nursing profession before the Ministry of Health.

Second, despite major changes in funding schemes for private clinics within the ever-expanding health market, wages for nurses in the public system remained unattractive and fixed within strict categories.[85] Although a legal frame[86] facilitated the expansion of private health services, an economic crisis in 1982 made it impossible for all the reforms to take place before the very last weeks of the government of Pinochet.[87] The subsequent process would nonetheless reinforce the purely regulatory role of the State,[88] becoming ever more difficult to have direct negotiations with it.

And third, one of the traits Chilean nurses felt most sensitive about—their university-based training as the sole entry route for practice—was threatened, as the government attempted to open nursing (and other) programs in higher education institutions other than universities. A united movement of all the professional associations did not seem achievable in this respect, and therefore the Board of the Nursing Association started independent negotiations with representatives of the public education system. For example, a petition to the President of the High Council of the University of Chile, Alejandro Medina Lois, sent in 1981,[89] and another one to the Minister of Education, Mónica Madariaga, sent in 1983,[90] recommending exclusivity in the requirement of university-based training. However, the Board was to report to fellow nurses "no positive results."[91] In the same year, a similar request was presented before the Ministry of Health, which was again rejected, though this time the aim was to re-establish high-ranking positions for nurses in healthcare institutions across the country.[92]

Although fruitless, the results are insightful. In contrast to the spirit of the October strike in 1972, when hordes of health workers protested against reforms outside the Parliament, this time social movements did not enjoy the necessary freedom to make their voice heard. While physicians, dentists, and pharmacists continued to discuss openly wages, work schedules, and the elimination of obligatory membership with their associations with the government, nurses, midwives, and physiotherapists either did not appear in those discussions or stayed offstage. As the correspondence shows, instead of actively criticizing the core of the reforms, which were capitalist in nature, the Board largely focused strictly on the consequences that would affect the profession and decided to rely heavily on diplomatic relations with different State instances. They did struggle to safeguard the collective interests of the profession, yet no open official criticism to the new model of State—or even worse, to systematic cruelties toward fellow nurses—was heard on the part of the Board members.

Toward the late 1970s, a favorable change of winds had come, when professional associations felt they could abolish the restrictions imposed on them. By reading the editorial sections of the Nursing Association's trade magazine from 1976 through 1979, one comes to the understanding that even the rightist Board members seemed to regret[93] their choice of collaborating with the Military so closely without receiving anything in return for the profession. These excerpts may serve as an example.

[The current restructuring] provoked big changes in the healthcare structure, which affected negatively our profession and other disciplines [...] Along with the difficult economic situation of our fellows, low expectations and scant incentives have discouraged many nurses who are now looking for new horizons [...] The year of 1976 has been one of the most difficult ones this Directorate and the members of the Honourable Board have faced.[94]

> It is internationally recognised that the nursing profession is a resource upon which depend quality care services of a nation. However, in this country its influence on high politics and its participation in the decisions that affect it directly are poor. [Being left out] represents a conspiracy against the image and mystique of our profession, leading to frustration and desertion of many nurses.[95]

Meanwhile, resisting movements within nursing, too, saw a revival, most notably led by a left-wing group called the *Movimiento de Renovación Gremial*. This same group would significantly counter the Board's initial positioning, which reached more salience in 1984, when its members took office at the Santiago branch of the Association.

But fears of life-threatening consequences were latent and even intensified through anonymous phone calls aimed at different professional leads, including the ones at the *Movimiento de Renovación Gremial*.[96][97] Discourses were enticing, but persecution, media censorship and forced "disappearances" became a barrier that carried well into the 1980s. Both perceived and actual, this barrier for re-democratization of professional associations threatened legitimacy and effectiveness of any attempt of internal elections. There was much to say, but much more could not be said.

Through the 2-year door-to-door work of the democratically elected nurses sitting on the Santiago branch,[98] albeit still under Pinochet's frightening rule, the non-democratic era eventually came to an end with internal elections of the National Board in 1986[99],[100] (see Table 1). The status of the association itself had been lowered. However, the new Board presented a structured makeover plan for the profession, one that sought to reunite the nurses across the country and across worldviews, regain what had been lost, and resume negotiations for nursing careers. Expectedly though, the culmination of an era marks the beginning of a new one. In this case, a transition that would allow for a rather unusual distribution of power, for this was the first left-wing Board of the Chilean Nurses Association ever since its creation.[101]

Related Work

Few publications have focused on similar developments and events. However, we should like to discuss some exemplary works relating the cases of Brazil (1960s), Portugal (1940s–1970s) and Spain (1930s–1970s), for they offer important insights. The Cold War era had parallel repercussions in Chile and Brazil, and its development had striking similarities in the sequence

TABLE 1. List of Presents of the Chilean Nurses Association Between 1965 and 2010, and Their Political Position

Period	Name	Affiliation or sympathy	Position during the conflict
1965–1969	Marilia Fonseca Corrales	Christian Democratic Party. Formerly a radical sympathizer	Neutral
1969–1971	Marta Donoso Carrasco	No information	No information
1971–1976[a]	Sonia Garrido Ballerino	Conservative right	Supporter of the *coup d'état* and of the military regime. Withheld protection to nurses with active participation in politics from 1973 onwards
	Elizabeth Gudelhoeffer G. (Vice-President)	Independent, right wing minded Relative of high-ranking Generals of the Military	Appointed advisor of nursing of the military government in 1973
	Gladys Peake Guevara (General Secretary)[b]	Movement for National Unity (conservative right). Formerly a Socialist militant	Supporter of the military regime
1977–1978	Viviana Corrales	No information	Supporter of the military regime
	Gladys Peake Guevara (General Secretary)	See above	Active adherent of a movement for a renewed right-wing party
1978–1982	Carmen Oye González	No information	No information
1982–1984	Sonia Garrido Ballerino	See above	Supporter of the military regime
1984–1986	Elizabeth Gudelhoeffer	See above	Sympathetic to the military regime

| 1986–1990 | Patricia Talloni Valdés | Left-wing minded Coalition of Parties for Democracy (center–left) | Advocated democratic elections of the Board members. Favored re-affiliation and pluralism while the Association was the target of anony-mous threats |
| 1990–2010 | Gladys Corral Neira | Social Democratic Force (originat-ing in the Com-munist Party) | Circulated position state-ments denouncing forced disappearances and filed lawsuits for homicides |

[a]From 1973 (*coup d'état*) to 1986 (when professional associations were allowed to hold meetings) the Board members were government-designated.
[b]Appointed permanently as either General Secretary or Vice-President or Regional Counsellor or Regional President or Editor of the trade magazine.

of events, in the sociopolitical ambience it created and in the intended pur-poses. President João Goulart of Brazil, who was neither a communist nor a revolutionary, assumed the presidency in 1961, following on from the former president's resignation. Critiques were that his thinking, as well as his policies, was compatible with communist ideals, which triggered his defeat in 1964. With the military in power, neoliberal reforms produced what came to be known as an "economic miracle," a discourse that reinforced the reform of the State but disguised human right violations—that is, a forceful integra-tion of Brazil into the international capitalist economy. As reforms reached the healthcare sector, the Board of the Brazilian Nurses Association expressed its willingness to "efficiently collaborate in the campaign for the develop-ment of the country," thinking that the sector needed drastic improvements. While there may, of course, be genuine reasons to support the Military techni-cally, the ideological assumptions beneath were soon questioned by dissident nurses. According to nurse historian Raimunda Medeiros Germano,[102,103] two divergent movements became apparent in the 1979 Nursing Congress held in Fortaleza. In the years thereafter, social movements intensified with ardent struggles for democracy,[104] with a sector of nurses creating a grouping called *Movimento Participação*[105,106] that would counter the hegemony of the Board members.[107] It has surfaced relatively recently that strong ties were kept be-tween rightist women of the United States, Chile, and Brazil, circulating flows of influence from and to those countries in their crusade against "godless" communism and the defence of moral values of the family[108]; although it is not certain whether nurses participated in those circles, it is very likely that at least the Board members shared information, correspondence and ideals, as some archives suggest.[109] The prominence of Chilean nurses in the Latin American healthcare,[110] along with their links with the Pan American Health Organization, US universities and, importantly, the Rockefeller Foundation, underscores this aspect as a worthy subject for further research. This would be important in understanding the flow and scope of influence. A key question would be, for example, where did the money for these activities come from? Granulating nurses' deployment of transnational activism would depict a much more complex image of professional women in the political sphere.

Although on a slightly different process but still within the international worldview dichotomy, António Salazar's dictatorship in Portugal is another case in point. It changed the usual model of mixed-gender nursing schools—in 1947 "a clear preference for female nursing students and subsequently for a female nursing staff"[111] was announced by law, which led to a subsequent shortage of nurses. Historian Helena da Silva states that this move was the result of an exaggerated view of the Anglo model of a nurse.[112] Interestingly, it is possible that Salazar also wanted to diminish the participation of nurses in politics by, mistakenly, feminizing the profession. By looking closely at the argument of the "natural" aptness of women for the care of the sick, we can infer that they were not considered a good fit for the political world, and would thus be more docile and instrumental in implementing administrative reforms. In fact, preexisting male nurses often gravitated toward—and even dominated—the Boards of the different nursing associations in Portugal, where female fellows could rarely sit.[113] Female nurses were considered most effective by the regime if they were unmarried, and on these grounds several nurses were persecuted; even one of them, who was also a militant of the *Movimento de Unidade Democrática* advocating for the right to be a married nurse and the workers' rights, was called "a communist" and eventually sentenced to prison until 1957.[114]

A similar case has been made for nurses working during the Francisco Franco era in Spain.[115] Fighting anti-monarchy groups, Franco's battle became an anti-communist stance, which in the process helped overcome the isolation of the Spanish economy. Two differing forces were dividing Spain: a liberal, democratic, reformist, pro-republic majority, and a nationalist, Catholic, anti-liberal minority.[116] By the time the Civil War broke out (1936), the military, the monarchy and the church had consolidated a vertical arrangement that seemed to give stability to the Spanish society in a climate of increasing labor mobilization and mistrust toward democratic institutions,[117] which caused the defeat of the 8-year-long democratically elected government (known as the Second Republic). As far as nursing was concerned, the romanticized and idealized image of women in society was centered on values such as children, home and church, a trilogy that made nurses fit in the broader cultural politics. In this value frame, the natural place of the woman was the family, while morality was an important component of education for ladies, constantly reinforced though nursing textbooks.[118] As international influences affected internal politics, two results appear pertinent to this analysis: on the one hand, the increasing social unrest of the 1960s with which some nurses felt identified, and on the other hand, a period of increasing technologization of nursing training in the 1970s (late *Franquismo*). As reported recently, Spanish nurses organized public demonstrations and succeeded in their demands of moving nursing education to universities in 1977,[119] taking advantages of a larger movement for democratization of society and the conjunction offered by health reforms. Although we are not told more details of the process, the 7-year-long negotiation shows that nurses were able to foreground a plan for the development of the profession, to undertake industrial action publicly, and to endure slow progress toward their purposes.

By treating the cases of Portugal and Spain together, one realizes the extent to which nurses played an instrumental role in cultural politics in the crafting of modern nations. For the embedded core values with which women contributed to the national sentiment, and by extension, served as role models. Reactionary in different ways, groups of nurses that grew unhappy with the status quo of repressive regimes could instigate gradual transformations. However, this area can be further problematized.

Interestingly, Chilean nurses sitting on the National Board of their Association often resorted to political strategies such as placating the Military, stating publicly their (unilateral) sociopolitical commitment toward the regime and, to some extent, fear-mongering about insurgent nurses and maneuvering the success of rightist nurses with the cross-national image of Chilean nursing. Given the situation, resisting groups had no option other than obstructing processes, keeping information to themselves, and using persuasion while questioning the lawfulness of the dictatorial government. Comparatively, these may respectively be transhistorical political strategies. Yet, whichever assumption one may take for the case of nursing during other dictatorships in Latin America, or elsewhere, historiographical scholarship addressing these matters is simply scant.

Conclusion

This article traces back the response of Chilean nurses to changes in political regimes as well as the flows of power across decades, governments, and political leanings, focusing on the 1970–1986 timespan. Unlike reified views on women as perpetually powerless individuals and female professions as strictly apolitical groupings, we have illustrated how nurses actively bargained ways to the Parliament, developed networks, participated in political leverage, applied calculated machination, and exerted resistance to oppression during a period of great political, economic, and social upheaval. While this story demonstrates that nurses faced particular impediments in being recognized as political actors and gaining access to political space, these insights shed light on the agency of nurses as both a large healthcare profession and an important part of the professionally trained female workforce.

As the second half of the 20th century unfolded, larger national and international interests offered the setting in which nurses sought to protect their own collective interests. However, two opposing worldviews worked their way through the Chilean Nurses Association, and in the process fractured a relatively homogeneous political stance. The dynamics of power then became very intricate and complex, to the point that they are difficult to distinguish from those of established, male professions which usually had more salience in the public sphere. Nurses, in fact, suffered the aftermaths of their political partaking in the same way other large professions did (i.e. medical doctors, teachers, lawyers, and journalists), and their respective associations mirrored the convoluted 1970s and 1980s.

Generally, the transition from the conservative governments to socialism opened up room for a gender agenda across classes and professions. Conversely, with the transition toward a repressive regime, nurses saw themselves in a rare scenario. While they had benefitted from Allende's gender-oriented agenda, paradoxically the professions' battle against Marxism led to an incredibly high participation of nurses joining the various confederations of professionals. This offered practice nurses a scenario where they could learn how to bargain by exerting many forms of industrial action. While the third transition covered in the manuscript is only addressed partially, the aftermaths of the military regime for nurses seem sharp. One is the attribution of the Association; since professional bodies were cast out of the state structure, their authority is scant—they have no control over the professionals, while professionals themselves are regulated by law and judged directly by the Court in case of infringement. Another one is the opening of a private market for nurses; once negatively perceived by nurses as some sort of "privatization of nursing," both private hospitals and private universities are now an important source of wages for nurses in Chile.

In the main, what this political history of Chilean nursing illustrates today is nurses' enduring tactics and devices with which to enter the political arena. In taking a stance in the values clash, nurses faced and responded to the State's underestimation, international criticism, third-party pressures, military oppression, and even other nurses' judgments. Although often referred to pejoratively as a dark era, examining this problematic period of history is useful in sifting significant findings that reverse the perception of women in public life and that of the female workforce in regard to the defence of their views.

Acknowledgments

We publicly recognize the help of the Chilean Nurses Association, the National Library of Chile, the Manuscripts and Archives service at Yale University Library, the Library of the Ministry of Health, the Library of the Chilean Medical Association, the International Council of Nursing, the Library and Archive Service of the Royal College of Nurses (UK), anonymous senior faculty nurses, former nurse leads, and family members of nurses who have passed on; especial thanks go to Francisca Aguirre Guedelhoefer. For edifying conversations and detailed feedback, we must thank Rafael Pedemonte (Ghent University) and Bernardo Alarcón (Université de Liège). For methodological inspiration, we are forever indebted to Margaret Power (Illinois Institute of Technology).

Comments by anonymous reviewers certainly helped us improve our manuscript and we express our gratitude to them. We also wish to recognize Lorena Bettancourt (University of Valparaiso) and Nancy Retamal (Catholic University of Chile) for assisting with copies of important archival materials. Finally, we acknowledge the support of Konrad Adenauer Foundation in providing a travel grant to one of the listed authors.

Notes

1. Permissions to publish excerpts from the interview transcripts were provided in writing by all interviewees. Interviews are stored at the University of Santiago School of Nursing.

2. Chile is a former colony of the Spanish Empire. Beginning in the early 19th century, the post-independence era witnessed increasing consolidation of a heavily centralised State, dominated by conservative ideas in creating a republican social order, though relying on international relations for commerce, population, and exploitation of the land for most of the century. Following on from the second industrial revolution (1880s), the State adopts an active role in redistributing the profits of international trade, which would eventually become social welfare policies from the (1920s) onwards. Along with Europe-inspired philanthropic oligarchy, close collaboration with international altruistic organizations created services that gave rise to a range of charity institutions and the National Health Service in the (1950s). Social reforms were increasingly questioned as the Cold War unfolded.

3. Elizabeth Rocío Núñez, "Enfermeras Chilenas (1970–1980): Dos décadas de transformación de la identidad, un legado para la memoria" (PhD diss., Andrés Bello National University, 2012).

4. Ricardo Ayala & Elizabeth Rocío Núñez, "Dusting off the looking-glass: A historical analysis of the development of a nursing identity in Chile," *Nursing Inquiry 24*, no. 1 (2017).

5. Ibid.

6. Margaret Power, "Who but a Woman? The Transnational Diffusion of Anti-Communism among Conservative Women in Brazil, Chile and the United States during the Cold War," *Journal of Latin-American Studies 47*, no. 1 (2015).

7. Marcela Cornejo, Francisca Mendoza and Rodrigo C. Rojas, "Research with Life Stories: Clues and Options," *Psyche 17*, no. 1 (2008).

8. Kate Murphy. "Feminism and Political History," *Australian Journal of Politics & History 56*, no. 1 (2010).

9. Richard Quantz, "Interpretive Method in Historical Research: Ethnography Reconsidered," in *The Teacher's Voice: A Social History of Teaching in Twentieth Century America*, ed. Richard J. Altenbaugh (London: Falmer Press, 1992), 174–94.

10. More than ever, Santiago became a different kind of Chile, an urban area with a relatively developed infrastructure and health care system, compared to the rest of the country. Thereby the focus on documentation produced in the capital reflects the over representation of the nurses working in metropolitan hospitals and of the Chilean Nurses Association, which was also based in the capital.

11. Eduardo Frei Montalva, "Primer mensaje del Presidente de la República de Chile, Don Eduardo Frei Montalva: al inaugurar el período de sesiones ordinarias del Congreso Nacional," Speech given at the National Congress, Santiago, (1965), Departamento de Publicaciones de la Presidencia de la República.

12. Eduardo Frei Montalva, "Segundo mensaje del Presidente de la República de Chile, Don Eduardo Frei Montalva: al inaugurar el período de sesiones ordinarias del Congreso Nacional," Speech given at the National Congress, Santiago, (1966), Departamento de Publicaciones de la Presidencia de la República.

13. Rosalba Flores, *Historia de la Enfermería en Chile* (Santiago: Universidad de Chile, 1965).

14. Hackett, June 26, 1941, Diaries.

15. Anonymous, e-mail message to authors (February 20, 2017).

16. Ibid., Hackett, (June 26, 1941).

17. Felícitas Klimpel, *La Mujer Chilena. El aporte femenino al progreso de Chile* (Santiago: Andrés Bello, 1962).

18. Yazmín Lecourt, "Relaciones de género y liderazgo de mujeres dentro del Partido Comunista de Chile" (Master diss., University of Chile, 2005).

19. David S. Parker and Louise E. Walker, *Latin America's Middle Class. Unsettled Debates and New Histories* (Lanham, MD: Lexington Books, 2013).

20. Norberto Espinoza, "Discurso de apertura IV Congreso Nacional de Enfermería de Valdivia [Speech given at the 4th National Congress of Nurses in Valdivia]," *Enfermería* 1, no. 6 (1965).

21. Alejo Lira Infante, "Chile entero le dará la mayoría absoluta," *El Diario Ilustrado*, (September 3, 1970), 1, http://www.memoriachilena.cl/archivos²/pdfs/MC0055788.pdf.

22. As stated in the archives of the National Parliament, the main instigators were Deputies R. Vives (Liberal Party), H. Ahumada (Radical Party), J.S. Correa (Conservative Party) and H. Bolados (Traditionalist Conservative Party). See, for example, the history of the law no. 11161 that creates the Chilean Nurses Association.

23. Bernardino Bravo Lira, "El movimiento asociativo en Chile (1924–1973)," *Separata de la Revista Política*, (1982).

24. William C. Davis, *Warnings from the Far South: Democracy versus Dictatorship in Uruguay, Argentina, and Chile* (Westport, CT and London: Praeger, 1995).

25. Margaret Power, *La mujer de derecha. El poder femenino y la lucha contra Salvador Allende*, 1964–1973 (Santiago: Centro de Investigaciones Barros Arana, 2008).

26. Ivonne Berliner, "Chilenas de Sectores Medios con Valores Conservadores Como Sujetos Políticos: (1964–1989)" (PhD diss., Universidad de Chile, Santiago).

27. Oral testimony, Retired nurse and former President of the Nurses Association.

28. Asociación de Enfermeras de Chile, "Cargo de enfermera sanitaria creado por el señor Ministro de Salubridad, el Doctor Salvador Allende, en el Valle del Choapa," *Boletín de la Asociación de Enfermeras de Chile* 1, no. 1 (1941).

29. Joseph Novitski, "Chile Restores Formal Ties with Cuba; End of Alignment with U.S. Policy Seen," *New York Times* (November 13, 1970), 2.

30. Salvador Allende, "Discurso en el Día Internacional de la Mujer." Speech given at Antofagasta, March 8, 1972.

31. Alfredo Jadresic, "La Facultad de Medicina durante el gobierno de la Unidad Popular," in *Salvador Allende. Presencia en la ausencia*, ed. Miguel Lawner, Hernán Soto and Jacobo Schatana (Santiago: LOM, 2008), 273–280.

32. Luis Corvalán, *El Gobierno de Salvador Allende* (Santiago: LOM, 2003).

33. National Congress of Chile, *Debates*, ordinary session no. 63, August 28, 1973.

34. National Congress of Chile, *Debates*, extraordinary session no. 73, September 3, 1973.

35. *El Mercurio* newspaper read on September 5, 1973: "The Chilean Nurses Association agreed in an assembly yesterday on continuing the strike for another 48 hours. The industrial action of these professionals aims to being included in Act 15076 On [medical] professional public servants."

36. *El Mercurio* newspaper read on September 5, 1973: "Stores Close. A Million Workers on Strike."

37. Chamber of Representatives, *Debates*, ordinary session no. 22, August 17, 1971.

38. Margaret Power, *Right-wing women in Chile: Feminine Power and the Struggle against. Allende* (University Park, PA: The Pennsylvania State University Press, 2002).

39. Sara Navas et al., *Testimony of the Chilean Female Professionals about the Change of Government* (Santiago: Editora Nacional Gabriela Mistral, 1973)

40. Guillermo Campero, *Los gremios empresariales en el período* (1970–1973). *Comportamiento sociopolítico y orientaciones ideológicas* (Santiago: Instituto Latinoamericano de Estudios Transnacionales, 1984).

41. The Allende administration lasted for about 3 years, suffering increasingly from inflation, interventionism, and speculation. A great portion of society—notably the professional workforce, industry owners, and centre–right and rightist parties—repeatedly asked President S. Allende to surrender and eventually demanded intervention of the armed forces. The *coup d'état* took place on September 11, 1973, during which circumstances the Presidential Palace was besieged by the Military and Allende's corpse taken out by soldiers. Recent official investigations delivered the finding that S. Allende committed suicide.

42. Luis Alvarez Baltierra, "Gremialismo. De la resistencia al desarrollo," *Ercilla*, no. 1991 (1973).

43. Oral testimony, Senior Nurse and former lead at a regional association of nurses.

44. American Embassy in Santiago to US Department of State, May 21, 1976.

45. American Embassy in Santiago to US Department of State, May 26, 1978.

46. Ibid. American Embassy, 1976.

47. Navas et al., *Testimony of the Chilean Female Professionals*, 6.

48. Sonia Garrido and Gladys Peake, "Carta enviada al General Augusto Pinochet U., Presidente de la Honorable Junta de Gobierno,"*Boletín Informativo 3*, no. 34–35–36 (1973).

49. Sonia Garrido and Gladys Peake, "A continuación damos a conocer la respuesta del General Don Augusto Pinochet U., Presidente de la Honorable Junta de Gobierno," *Boletín Informativo 3*, no. 34–35–36 (1973).

50. Rosalba Flores, "Editorial," *Boletín Informativo 3*, no. 34–35–36 (1973).

51. Junta Nacional de Gobierno, *Primer año de la Reconstrucción Nacional* (Santiago: Gabriela Mistral, 1974), http://www.memoriachilena.cl/602/w3-article-65341.html.

52. Sonia Garrido, "El Colegio de Enfermeras informa al mundo acerca de la situación nacional," *Boletín Informativo del Colegio de Enfermeras 3*, no. 34–35–36 (1973).

53. Colegio de Enfermeras de Chile, "Algunas noticias que Ud. debe conocer," *Enfermería* 29 (1971).

54. Asesoría Sra. Lidia Díaz para el Dr. Juricic T., Bogoslov, Ministry of Health, Department of International Affairs (February 26, 1975). Archivo Nacional de Administración, Documentos (1932–1991) (Doc. 1896-0419). Archives of Ministerio de Salud, Santiago de Chile.

55. Chilean Nurses Association. Notice No. 63, on the increase of nurses' working hours (October 1973).

56. Oral testimony, Senior Nurse.

57. For example, Gladys Peake, appointed Head of the Nursing Division at the NHS from 1971 onwards; and Betty Gudelhoefer, Advisor of Vice-Secretary of Health Commander Angel Guzmán Veliz, from 1973 to 1976.

58. Oral testimony, Senior Nurse.

59. Mª Eugenia Somalo, "Congreso de Tokio. Tema del día 3 de Junio de (1977)," *Boletín Cultural e Informativo del Consejo General de Ayudantes Técnicos Sanitarios* (1978).

60. Professional Associations Act, L. 3261 (1981).

61. Oral testimony, Senior Nurse-Midwife.

62. Corporación Nacional de Reparación y Reconciliación. *Informe de la Comisión Nacional de Verdad y Reconciliación. Informe Rettig, 2nd ed.* (Santiago: Andros, 1996). http://www.memoriachilena.cl/archivos2/pdfs/MC0053679.pdf.

63. Colegio de Enfermeras de Chile, "Juramento Internacional," *Enfermería 39* (1974).

64. International Committee of the Red Cross. Report on the visit of the delegate-general for Latin America to Chile. *Annual report 1973* (1974): 32–40.

65. Amnesty International, *Annual Report* (1973–1974) (London: Amnesty International Publications, 1974).

66. See the (1975) International Council of Nurses' position statement: "The Nurse's Role in the Care of Detainees and Prisoners."

67. Agrupación de Familiares de Ejecutados Políticos, "Día Internacional de la mujer: Homenaje a las mujeres asesinadas por la dictadura" (1990): 6.

68. Chilean Nurses Association *v.* General Augusto Pinochet (September 14, 1998).

69. The most infamous cases were those of Gladys Corral, Margarita Reusch, Patricia Talloni, Celsa Parrau, Patricia Grau, Miriam Bergholz, Hortensia Arizabala and Patricia Herrero, but after the transition to democracy—in 1990—it has surfaced that very many other nurses in all regions were also affected and worked under political repression. In a press release in (1988), the Association stated, "We really did not want to make these incidents known because we do not want to let them [the Military] threaten our colleagues."

70. Private hospitals were most often dominated by right-wing owners, and nurses had no private income source.

71. Former leaders of professional associations, "Colegios profesionales y asociaciones gremiales durante el proceso de recuperación de la democracia en Chile," interview by Gabriel Guzmán, *Report of the Museo de la Memoria y los Derechos Humanos*, June 12, 2012, 91.

72. Former leaders of professional associations, interview, 97.

73. Juanita Rojas, "Requeridos: por el delito de opinar," *Análisis 9*, no. 135 (1986).

74. Sonia Garrido and Glays Peake, "Posición del Colegio de Enfermeras frente a las Colegiadas Funcionarias Cuestionadas," *Boletín Informativo 3*, no. 34–35–36 (1973).

75. Oral testimony, senior faculty nurse.

76. Oral testimony, senior community nurse.

77. Jorge Chuaqui, Lorena Bettancourt and Valentina Leal, "Contexto social y gremial como aspectos de la identidad en Enfermería," in *XXIX Congress of the Latin-American Sociological Association*, ed. ALAS. Santiago: ALAS (2013).

78. There were those who justified the economy switch but not the dictatorship, those who supported military intervention as a transitory measure for social order only, those who encouraged social order but not at the expense of human rights, those who were UP supporters but did not exculpate it from the crisis, and so on.

79. Jaime Llambias-Wolff, *The Rise and Fall of Welfare Health Legislation in 20th Century Chile. A Case Study in Political Economy of Law* (York University, Canada, 2014).

80. Alison J. Bruey, "Limitless Land and the Redefinition of Rights: Popular Mobilization and the Limits of Neoliberalism in Chile (1973–1985)," *Journal of Latin American Studies 44*, no. 3 (2012).

81. Llambias-Wolff, *The Rise and Fall*, 175–176.

82. Manuel Annick, "El sistema de salud chileno: 20 años de reformas," *Salud Pública de México* 2 (2002).

83. Modelos de Atención de Enfermería by Alicia Cartes Aguilera, Sofía Matus Lagos and Lidia Díaz for Ministry of Health, Department of Nursing Programs Support (1979). (Doc. 1–28). Archives of the Museo Nacional de la Medicina, Santiago de Chile.

84. Llambias-Wolff, *The Rise and the Fall*, 63.

85. Encasillamiento By Dr. Hector Concha Marambio, Ministry of Health. Central Comission of Restructuring (October 15, 1979). Archivo Nacional de Administración, Documentos (1932–1991) (Doc. 2008–2031), Archives of Ministerio de Salud, Santiago de Chile.

86. Health Services and Benefits Act, L. 03 (1981).

87. Creation of the Superintendence of Health Act, L. 18933 (1981).

88. Manuel Annick, *El sistema de salud chileno*, 63.

89. Colegio de Enfermeras de Chile, "Editorial," *Enfermería* 67 (1981).

90. Colegio de Enfermeras de Chile, "Editorial," *Enfermería* 77 (1983).

91. Ibid.

92. Ibid.

93. Especially in the pieces entitled: "Clarinada de Advertencia," "Sistema de Unidad Operativa de Salud," "Los Colegios Profesionales," "Perspectivas y Realidades."

94. Chilean Nurses Association, "Editorial. 25 años del Colegio de Enfermeras (1953–1978). Memoria Anual del Consejo General del Colegio de Enfermeras de Chile," *Enfermería* 12 (1978): 33.

95. Chilean Nurses Association, "Editorial. Clarinada de Advertencia," *Enfermería*, 12 (1978): 3.

96. Juanita Rojas, "Colegio de Enfermeras: Defender la salud, defender la profesión," *Análisis* (1988): 20.

97. Anonymous. "El amedrentamiento volvió al Colegio de Enfermeras." *Fortín Mapocho* (February 13, 1988). http://www.archivomuseodelamemoria.cl/uploads/1/8/188254/00000617000003000008.pdf.

98. Nurses for Unity and Democracy Group (1986), *Informativo*, pamphlet.

99. Anonymous, "Triunfo opositor en Colegio de Enfermeras," *Análisis* 155 (1986).

100. Consejo Regional Santiago, "Tras un democrático proceso electoral. Nuevas Directivas en el Colegio de Enfermeras," *Revista del Consejo Regional Santiago* 8 (1986).

101. Ibid. Ricardo Ayala and E. Rocío Núñez, "Dusting off the looking-glass."

102. Raimunda Medeiros Germano, "Percurso revisitado: o ensino de enfermagem no Brasil," *Pro-Posições 14*, no. 1 (2003).

103. Raimunda Germano Medeiros, *A Ética e o Ensino de Ética na Enfermagem do Brasil*" (São Paulo: Cortez, 1993).

104. Érica Toledo de Mendonça, "Enfermagem-Saúde: construindo um saber sobre políticas de saúde, 1977–1980" (Master diss., Universidade Federal do Estado do Rio De Janeiro, 2009).

105. Maria José dos Santos Rossi, "A propósito do movimento participação," *Revista Brasileira de Enfermagem 54*, no. 2 (2001).

106. Gelson Luiz de Albuquerque and, Denise Elvira Pires de Pires, "O movimento participação (MP): uma contribuição à história da enfermagem brasileira," *Revista Brasileira de Enfermagem 54*, no. 2 (2001).

107. Ibid. Raimunda Medeiros Germano, "Percurso revisitado."

108. Ibid. Margaret Power, "Who but a Woman?

109. Mary Ann Menezes Freire, "Levantamento de Recursos e Necessidades de Enfermagem no Brasil: da pesquisa ao livro (1956–1980)" (Master diss., Universidade Federal do Estado do Rio De Janeiro, 2011).

110. Apart from the stated facts, the perception of the interviewees was that "Chilean nurses worked closely with PAHO and that they contributed to create the majority of the nursing schools in Latin America." Oral testimony.

111. Helena da Silva, "Being a male nurse in Portugal during Salazar's dictatorship (1940–1970)," *Nursing Inquiry 20*, no. 2 (2013): 176–185, 179

112. Ibid. Helena da Silva, "Being a male nurse in Portugal."

113. Ibid.

114. Helena da Silva, "Selecção e discriminação dos profissionais de enfermagem durante o Estado Novo (1938–1963)," *Ler História* 60, (2011).

115. Margalida Miró, Denise Gastaldo, Sioban Nelson and Gloria Gallego, "Spanish Nursing under Franco: Reinvention, Modernization and Repression (1956–1976)," *Nursing Inquiry 19*, no. 3 (2012).

116. Luis Alberto Romero, "La Guerra Civil Española y la polarización ideológica y política: la Argentina 1936–1946," *Anuario Colombiano de Historia Social y de la Cultura 38*, no. 2 (2011).

117. Claudio Hernández Burgos, "Las Bases Sociales de la dictadura y las Actitudes Ciudadanas Durante el Régimen de Franco. Granada (1936–1976)" (PhD diss., University of Granada, 2012).

118. Ibid. Margalida Miró, Denise Gastaldo, Sioban Nelson and Gloria Gallego, "Spanish nursing under Franco."

119. Ibid.

RICARDO A. AYALA, PhD
Department of Sociology
Ghent University
Korte Meer 3-5, B-9000 Gent, Belgium

MARKUS THULIN
Department of Iberian and Latin-American History
University of Cologne
Albertus-Magnus-Platz, D-50931 Cologne, Germany

E. ROCÍO NÚÑEZ, PhD
School of Nursing
University of Santiago
Av Bernardo O'Higgins 3363, 9160000 Estación Central
RM Santiago, Chile

FESTSCHRIFT FOR SUSAN REVERBY

Introduction

MERLIN CHOWKWANYUN
Columbia University

It is an honor to introduce pieces commemorating Susan Reverby's scholarship, mentorship, and activism. The pieces highlight several dimensions of her career that are worth discussing as a whole at the outset. Chief among them is the breadth of Susan's work. We often bemoan specialization in the academy and look for examples of those who have transcended it. Susan is one such person. Besides the history of nursing, she has made signal contributions to the historical study of women and gender, social movements, race and racism, labor, and medicine and public health. Indeed, a typical Reverby's article or book contains a holism that engages two or more of these fields at the same time: conceptualizing nursing within the larger political economy of work; situating Tuskegee within larger hereditarian narratives about the supposed biology of race; and more recently, analyzing masculinity, political violence, and the milieu of 1960s radicalism in her forthcoming biography of activist Alan Berkman.

For most, these accomplishments would be satisfying enough—and then some. But Susan has played a second critical role as well: mentor to generations of graduate and undergraduate students who have sought her advice, including all of the people participating in this symposium. I have encountered many of Susan's former Wellesley students who tell me about the impact her classes had on how they think and on their careers, whether in academia, the healing professions, law, social services, or whatever else. Then, there are people like myself just 5 years ago: the dozens of graduate students and junior scholars whose work Susan read and to whom she gave critical

Nursing History Review 27 (2019): 87–90. A Publication of the American Association for the History of Nursing. Copyright © 2019 Springer Publishing Company.
http://dx.doi.org/10.1891/1062-8061.27.87

pep talks, especially when the going became rough. Although Susan has often served formally on dissertation committees, much of her mentorship is silent and uncredited because Wellesley is not a PhD-granting institution. This lack of credit is outrageous! My hope is that this symposium serves as a corrective and tribute to her enormous generosity.

Finally, there is Susan's political engagement. Her scholarship successfully walks a taut line. There's always an eye toward social injustice in our present world. But there's another one that looks at how historical analysis might shed light on and even counteract it. With enormous care and introspection, Susan has balanced these imperatives. As she completed *Examining Tuskegee*, we spent hours on the phone and at conferences debating how to render various historical subjects responsibly and how to apply ethical and moral standards in hindsight. What was the difference between apologia for racism versus analyzing people's actions according to the institutional and cultural norms of the time? How could one assign deserved blame while at the same time not just depicting Tuskegee as just another episode of unremitting racism in American medicine?[1] With her Berkman biography, Susan is wrestling with the same issues. Her subject is simultaneously sympathetic, naïve, reckless, and heroic, sometimes at the same moment.

For junior scholars and graduate students, the care with which Susan approaches historical writing is a model. And so in closing, I'd like to share briefly my personal experience with Susan's kindness and encouragement toward those much lower on the pecking order. I first met her more than a decade ago. I was a 21-year-old undergraduate with intermittent bathing and sleeping habits, and I got in touch with her to interview her as a historical subject. Susan was a member of an activist research collective in New York City called the Health/Policy Advisory Center (Health/PAC), which published a *Bulletin* that critically analyzed health issues from a left-wing perspective. The common thread linking all of Susan's reminiscence was one that she confronted repeatedly as a scholar: how to marry political goals with honest analysis? Her answer in our conversation was there (a) wasn't a single recipe to do so and (b) harmonizing both would probably always occur less than ideally. One story sticks out: Susan recalled submitting an article on abortion, only to be told by another member of Health/PAC that the piece was flawed because it "didn't fit the [Health/PAC] framework." A priori ideology, in other words, was trumping empirical fidelity. Enough experiences like these eventually sent Susan back to graduate school, even though she has hardly eschewed political engagement since.

I kept in touch with Susan after the interview. When I began graduate school at the University of Pennsylvania, Susan organized a panel where I delivered my first conference paper at the American Association for the History of Medicine's Sigerist Circle, a sub-section (some might say refuge) for lefty historians. In subsequent years, she regularly checked in on me to see how I was doing and lent an ear when things weren't going well, which was more often than I care to remember. As she did with others like myself, she line-edited drafts, wrote letters of recommendation for me, and let me gab and gripe, even though she had zero formal obligation to do so and never served in any official advisory capacity. When I needed to research at the Countway Library of Medicine in Cambridge, Massachusetts, where Susan and her partner Bill Quivers live, she converted her house into what I affectionately called Hotel Reverby and let me stay with them for free (a commonality noted in Fairman's essay).

Above all, I most appreciate Susan's treatment of myself and others in my peer group as equals. I don't mean "equals" in the sense that she pretends we know as much or more than she does. I certainly don't now and certainly didn't then, when I first met her a decade ago. What I mean, however, is that Susan cares about our maturation as scholars; reveals to us her own scholarly struggles and doubts; and solicits our views on issues (including when they might diverge from hers). "Why would she care what I think?" I recall asking myself, the first time Susan asked me to read one of her manuscripts. Looking back, though, her asking meant a lot to me. It was her belief that I had something of value to say, and it gave me a critical psychic lift to continue doing the work. As a teacher myself now, I see that the best pedagogy is dialectical and two-way; Susan is one of the major people in my life who helped me see this.

When Susan told me about her intention to retire, I was initially sad. However, in her e-mail signature, Susan notes, with typical wry Reverby humor, that she has simply been "Repurposed and Not Retired." Is this an ironic nod to human resources babble (Susan has a bachelor's degree in "labor and industrial relations" that she routinely mocks)? Or is it her declaration that nothing's really changed? Probably a bit of both. But definitely the latter, if her prodigious output in the past couple years is any indication. I, for one, am sure glad that we will enjoy Susan's brilliant scholarly contributions and giving spirit for years more to come!

Note

1. Susan wrestles with these reviews in an incredibly astute critical reading of Harriet Washington's *American Apartheid: The Dark History of Medical Experimentation*

on Black Americans from Colonial Times to the Present. See Susan Reverby, "Inclusion and Exclusion: The Politics of History, Difference, and Medical Research," *Journal of the History of Medicine and Allied Sciences* 63, no. 1 (December 2007): 103–113.

MERLIN CHOWKWANYUN, MPH, PHD
Mailman School of Public Health
Columbia University
722 West 168th St. #R931
New York, NY 10034

Finding Susan Reverby

Julie A. Fairman
University of Pennsylvania

This is a personal story about friendship, mentorship, and scholarly tensions that shaped the discipline of the history of nursing.[1] I am one of the beneficiaries of that legacy. In 1985, I began my graduate program at the University of Pennsylvania mentored by a wonderful trio of historians, Joan Lynaugh, Karen Buhler-Wilkerson, and Ellen Baer, who introduced me to Susan Reverby's work. She had recently published her groundbreaking book, *Ordered to Care: The Dilemma of American Nursing, 1850–1945*, and I was struck by her ability to capture the history of the nursing profession beyond the frame of nursing victimhood.[2] She seemed to understand the profession's history, which I learned was in part though her intellectual relationships with Buhler-Wilkerson, Lynaugh, and Baer. I was also inspired by her skill connecting the history of nursing to larger social issues of the time, which directed me in my later work in the history of nursing and health policy. In this article, I will share how some historians of nursing "found" Susan Reverby (and how she found us!), how they shaped each other's work, and then situate this story as a way to think about the future of the discipline of the history of nursing.

This is, of course, a story from my own perspective, and I acknowledge it will not be everyone's story or describe a universal experience in the history of nursing. For example, the graduate students I have mentored might be hearing this for the first time and may or may not make the same historiographic connections. There will be gender, class, and race differences of experience, as nurses researching the history of nursing were a privileged group. Their identity as primarily white women academics shaped their questions and the sources they used. There is also a difference of place, as scholars in other areas across the country were studying the history of nursing. Nonetheless, this will, perhaps, help situate the historiography of the history of nursing as a place for lively and important debates about its current status and its future directions.

Nursing History Review 27 (2019): 91–98. A Publication of the American Association for the History of Nursing. Copyright © 2019 Springer Publishing Company.
http://dx.doi.org/10.1891/1062-8061.27.91

This particular story focuses on how Reverby, Buhler-Wilkerson, Lynaugh, and Baer found each other and sketched an ambitious agenda (although none of them would say this was a formal plan) for developing and sustaining the history of nursing as a legitimate, scholarly, and interdisciplinary field. They envisioned training nurses as historians to create a discipline separate from although tied to the history of medicine, and finally, to convince historians in other disciplines to situate nursing as a way to think differently about their own historical work. They believed that medical, labor, women's, and gender history, and history of technology would necessarily be broadened and resituated by locating nurses as part of the historical narrative, and that nurses with training in historical scholarship could provide critical perspectives to those in other disciplines.

Although this story is somewhat serendipitous, as history is wont to be, it also illuminates underpinnings that shaped the thinking of Buhler-Wilkerson, Lynaugh, and Baer in the direction of interdisciplinarity, as well as the importance of developing intellectual and personal relationships through common scholarly and activist interests. Both factors were foundational for the developing field of the history of nursing. Crucially, Buhler-Wilkerson, Lynaugh, and Baer all completed their graduate and postgraduate work mentored by historians.[3] All three believed that if nurses were to be part of a growing body of research focused on the history of medicine, health, and illness, and on those who provided care, they had to forge interdisciplinary links with scholars outside their professional schools, as they did. There were few other historians of nursing in schools of nursing who could provide support and mentorship.

Although graduate education in history shaped Buhler-Wilkerson, Lynaugh, and Baer's disciplinary approach, their introduction to Susan Reverby, and the intellectual and personal relationships that formed came unexpectedly. They were, however, a critical ingredient that shaped the discipline. When Buhler-Wilkerson was a graduate student at The University of Pennsylvania (Penn) in the early 80s, her work on public health nurses took her to the American Nurses Association (ANA) and the Association of Public Health Nursing archives at the Howard Gotlieb Archives Research Center, Mugar Memorial Library, Boston University. On a previous trip, Buhler-Wilkerson stayed at the YWCA to save money. But her mentor, Charles Rosenberg, suggested she contact Reverby to find better accommodations, as she lived in Boston. I speculate he also believed they would find shared interests. Reverby quickly invited Buhler-Wilkerson to stay with her, which became a long-standing tradition. Buhler-Wilkerson found Reverby to be an interested and expert reader of her work, and both found commonalities in their feminist and activist views. Buhler-Wilkerson then introduced Lynaugh and Baer to Reverby as someone who could and wanted to support their work to shape the history of nursing discipline. In turn, Buhler-Wilkerson, Lynaugh, and Baer also read and critiqued Reverby's work on the history of nursing. It became a two-way intellectual relationship.

Reverby was familiar with nursing as a subject, as she had been writing about health professions, including nursing, since the early 1970s. Her undergraduate degree in industrial relations and labor history from Cornell University (1967), as well as her MA in American Civilization from New York University (1973), created a foundation for her work on nursing from an activist feminist and labor history perspective. In the 1970s, she began contributing as a staff researcher and writer at Health/PAC, the Health Policy Advisory Center, which was a private liberal policy advocacy center in New York City.[4] As part of her research for her writings, she read the *American Journal of Nursing* and discovered a kindred spirit in Lavinia Dock, a nurse, social activist, and feminist. Her pieces for the *Health/Pac Bulletin* channeled Dock's activism on behalf of women and women health workers. Her writings included pieces such as the "Sorcerer's Apprentice,"[5] about the newly emerging roles of physician assistants and nurse practitioners, and "Health: Women's work,"[6] which focused on the hierarchy and unequal division of labor in caregiving in and out of institutions. As the professional nursing world debated the 1964 ANA declaration of the BSN as the education entry point for nurses, Reverby already identified the class and ideological implications of a hierarchical nursing labor force that had not yet claimed its identity as a "thinking" profession that its leaders conceptualized.

Her work at Health/PAC and unanswered questions, as Kline notes in a separate essay in this issue, led Reverby to a PhD program at Boston University, where she initially set out to examine women's domestic service. She changed direction when the requirements of a grant opportunity with the Milbank Multidisciplinary Program, directed by sociologist John McKinely, coaxed her to focus on nursing and the power dynamics that shaped the profession and nurses' work within hospitals as a field of interest. She immersed herself in nursing archival sources not typically examined by other historians, and consulted with several practicing nurses, including Karen Buhler-Wilkerson, nursing alumni associations and their graduates.

Her dissertation in 1982, *The Nursing Disorder: A Critical History of the Hospital-Nursing Relationship, 1869–1945* (which she later revised as her book, *Ordered to Care*) shook the nursing discipline and profession. Rather than celebrating and documenting nursing leaders' efforts to advance nursing as a knowledge-based profession, she illustrated nursing leaders' inability to resolve the tensions between nurses' control over their own practice and hospitals' and physicians' attempts to control the nursing workforce. She pointed out the paradox of nurses' duty and obligation as women to care while also seeking training and wages.

Her treatment of nursing was in contrast to the celebratory- or victim-based analyses that had emerged from earlier nursing writers, such as nurse Joanne Ashley. Although Reverby believed Ashley's 1979 book, *Hospitals, Paternalism and the Role of the Nurse*,[7] was path-breaking because it took on sexism and economic paternalism (which appealed to many nursing leaders at the time), she also challenged Ashley's perception of nurses as subservient, powerless, and exploited by the sexism of physicians and systematic hospital paternalism.[8] Citing historian E.P. Thompson's writing on the limits of claiming paternalism as a monolithic force, Reverby drew on her archival sources and saw a more complicated and nuanced history.[9] As she noted, "Ashely failed to explain under what conditions accommodation yielded to resistance and noncooperation on the part of some, or why others actively saw accommodation as salvation."[10] Ashley, perhaps because of her own experiences as a nurse, "too harshly judged and blamed its [nursing's] past. Nurses are neither the poor victims of hospital and physician oppression and the impotent descendants of a long line of women healers, nor the victors in a difficult and long struggle to gain professional recognition and status."[11] As Reverby notes on the last page of her dissertation, "nursing's history should not be judged too harshly, but it should be understood."[12]

With their common interests in women's work, feminism, and nursing, Reverby, Buhler-Wilkerson, Lynaugh, and Baer were an effective quartet agitating for change and better historical understanding in an insular and conservative field. Reverby cautioned them to not only to encourage historical training but to support those clinicians who did not have it, which encompassed many nurses who wrote about the history of nursing. She reminded them that similar issues in the history of medicine had created in rift in the early 1980s between clinicians who were interested in history and historians (who were not clinicians) interested in medicine. These conflicts created hierarchies and tension in the American Association of the History of Medicine as historians began to outnumber clinicians. Reverby is a good example of someone who was trained as a historian but, through her training in history, and her activism and feminism, could also cross disciplines and interrogate power structures that operated in the nursing workplace and workforce. She also privileged the experience and knowledge of those who worked in institutions and with patients. As Joan noted, "we all wanted to be like Susan [Reverby]" and cross interdisciplinary boundaries.

Not everyone believed historians outside the profession could understand nursing and its history. The American Association for the History of Nursing (AAHN) (initially the International History of Nursing Society), founded in 1978, held its first meeting in 1984 in Charlottesville, VA. Buhler-Wilkerson and Lynaugh were part of the meeting planning group and arranged to have Reverby comment on a article at the meeting (historians Janet Golden and Susan Armeny also presented articles). As Reverby noted, "[the article she was asked to critique] was ahistoric—it was the kind of article that you wouldn't let get published or presented if it was your student." Her official remarks were more subtle, and she argued that there were many ways to think about the data the writer presented. She tried to be polite but she was perceived by many in the audience as an outside agitator.

I remember hearing about this meeting and how defensively many responded to Reverby's comments. One person in the audience began her approach with the rejoinder, "how dare you suggest..." with others raising similar questions. After the meeting, many of the historians who were not nurses saw the AAHN as an unfriendly venue for their work and stayed away from the organization for many years. Lack of exposure to interdisciplinary scholars left the field more insular and drove others to different organizations. Reverby continued to write about nurses, their power and their politics even as she moved on to other subjects, but she rarely participated in the AAHN meetings again.

Even so, this meeting stimulated other like-minded nurses to join Buhler-Wilkerson, Lynaugh, and Baer to strengthen the history of nursing, to seek training in historical methods and history in general, and to support and encourage interdisciplinary scholars. Reverby was part of a growing cadre of historians, such as Susan Armeny, Darlene Clark Hines, Nancy Tomes, and Barbara Melosh, who also saw nursing as an important way to analyze institutions, medicine and women's work, and interrogate race. Historians of nursing also began to unpack their own history as a way to better understand the complexity of its claims to advocacy, identity, knowledge, and their power within and outside of institutions.

As groups of historians came together at schools and colleges of nursing, they began to organize artifacts and other archival holdings to document the history of nursing.[13] By 1982, Buhler-Wilkerson, Lynaugh, and Baer conceptualized an intellectual space for scholars and students, as well as an archival repository that might attract interdisciplinary scholars. Supported by a substantial gift from nurse Lillian Brunner (the author of the best-selling, *Textbook of Medical Surgical Nursing*) and support from Penn Graduate Program Director Florence Downs, who favored dissertations in nursing history, the Center for the Study of the History of Nursing (eventually renamed The Barbara Bates Center for the Study of the History of Nursing, after physician Barbara Bates) opened in 1985. Claire Fagin, then the Dean of the School of Nursing at the University of Pennsylvania, was a key supporter and brought together a group of interdisciplinary scholars such as historians Reverby, Charles Rosenberg, Rosemary Stevens, and Villanova Dean and historian of nursing Louise Fitzpatrick and others, to provide intellectual guidance that was prescient and innovative for the time.

My fellow students—Patricia D'Antonio, Meryn Stewart, and later, Cynthia Connolly, Mary Ann Krisman Scott, Ann Marie Walsh Brennan, Jean Whalen—and I were very fortunate to be part of a new generation of history of nursing scholars mentored by nurse historians and grounded by historical inquiry. We were encouraged to cross disciplines and study with historians of labor, gender, science, medicine, and technology at Penn. But, our choices to conduct historical research would not be the easiest ones. Sometimes, other historians questioned our legitimacy as scholars. Sometimes, our nursing colleagues questioned the value of our methods and our work. Our confidence to continue in history came from a critical leap of faith by our mentors in our intellectual capabilities, as well as Reverby's acknowledgment of our work while role-modeling spirited critique and scholarly engagement.

As the field grew, we were also some of the earliest graduate students to be funded by NIH F31s and F32s, as well as through National Library of Medicine and National Endowment for the Humanities grants. Reverby wrote letters of support for us, reviewed our book proposals and manuscripts, served as an independent study advisor. We developed new connections with other historians, and they began to read our work and take on nursing as a lens for understanding broader historical questions. But even so, it was sometimes hard to be taken seriously by historians who "did not know us," a reflection on the historical continuity of the clinician/historian divide. Some historians saw us as their project, identifying us as marginalized and the victims of the medical hierarchy. Reverby helped us come to terms with our own power and to help us move beyond the victimization narratives that sometimes still surfaced. In turn, we influenced Reverby's work on the history of nursing through our own research, conversations, and critique.

Reverby found the history of nursing, and the history of nursing found Reverby. But where do we go from here? Have we become "like Susan?" And, can we empower our students as Reverby and our mentors empowered us? I have to think that my colleagues and I can support the intellectual growth of new generations. We do have students who have and are forging into new areas such as international studies, history of technology, Africana Studies, and women's studies. Our students have gone on to mentor others as we mentored them. And, many interdisciplinary scholars, to paraphrase historian Joan Scott, do see nursing as a useful category of historical analysis.[14]

Some continuity has sustained the collaborative environment of the 80s and 90s into the 21st century. Similar to the experiences of Kline and Chowkwanyun (in this issue), Reverby's interdisciplinary role-modeling, her generosity, activism, and support influenced our engagement with our students. Reverby helped us see that our history was more than the stories of the great men and women physicians, nurse leaders, or institutions. Our history was also about the women and men—the practicing nurses—who had enormous power with patients in institutions and in their communities, and who were a critical part of the success and failures of new therapeutics, research, models of care, and technology. She encouraged us to find meaning in these stories, to embrace the complexity of our intellectual challenges, and delight in our achievements over time, and at the same time, perhaps stir things up a bit. Our students and graduates have forged into new areas and new sources of support, gaining traction with a public and a profession thirsting for a clearer understanding of their options and place in our current health care environment. But, a great deal of creativity and new interdisciplinary engagement, as experienced by Buhler-Wilkerson, Lynaugh, and Baer with Reverby, will still be needed to support and encourage a new generation of scholars and their future successes in academic settings.

Acknowledgments

This article is based in part on informal conversations with Susan Reverby and Joan Lynaugh in Spring, 2017.

Notes

1. This article is an edited version of a panel presentation at the American Association of the History of Medicine, *Susan Reverby's Contributions to the History of Medicine, Public Advocacy, and the History of Nursing: A Roundtable* (May, 2017).

2. Susan Reverby, *Ordered to Care: The Dilemma of American Nursing* (1850–1945), Cambridge History of Medicine (Cambridge, Boston, MA: Cambridge University Press, 1987).

3. Lynaugh studied with historian John Burhnam at the Ohio State University, and Forest Berghorn, who was Chair of American Studies at the University of Kansas, but her dissertation advisor was historian Regina Morantz-Sanchez (completed in 1982). Buhler-wilkerson, although starting her studies in Urban Planning at Penn, also studied with historian Charles Rosenberg (also her dissertation chair, 1984), then at Penn, in the History and Sociology of Science Department. Baer studied at New York University with historian Paul Mattingly and philosopher Elizabeth Bridston, and completed her dissertation (1982) under nurse theorist Pat Winstead-Fry. She went on to post-doctoral research (1986) in social history funded by the National Center for Nursing Research (precursor to the National Institute of Nursing Research) and sponsored by historian Charles Rosenberg.

4. Merlin Chowkwanyun, "The New Left and Public Health The Health Policy Advisory Center, Community Organizing, and the Big Business of Health (1967–1975)," *American Journal of Public Health 101*, no. 2 (2011): 238–249.

5. Susan Reverby, "The Sorcerer's Apprentice," *HealthPac Bulletin*, November 1972, 10–16.

6. Susan Reverby, "Health: Women's Work," *HealthPac Bulletin*, April 1972, 15–20.

7. Jo Ann Ashley, *Hospitals, Paternalism, and the Role of the Nurse* (New York: Teachers College Press, 1979).

8. Susan Reverby, "Review of Joanne Ashley. Hospital, Paternalism, and the Role of the Nurse," *Social Science & Medicine 11*, no. 6–7 (April 1977).

9. E. P. Thompson, "Eighteenth Century English Society: Structure, Field-of-Force, Dialectic" (University of Pittsburgh, Department of History, 1976).

10. Susan Mokotoff Reverby, "The Nursing Disorder: A Critical History of the Hospital-Nursing Relatsionship (1860–1945)," xxv.

11. Susan Mokotoff Reverby, xxv.

12. Susan Mokotoff Reverby, "The Nursing Disorder: A Critical History of the Hospital-Nursing Relatsionship, 1860–1945" (Boston University, 1982), 376.

13. The University of Wisconsin Milwaukee, College of Nursing, Center for Nursing History had been collecting artifacts and the papers of selected individuals since (1975). The Center for Historical Inquiry in Nursing, recently renamed the Eleanor Crowder Bjoring Center for Nursing Historical Inquiry, opened in 1991.

14. Joan W. Scott, "Gender: A Useful Category of Historical Analysis," *The American Historical Review 91*, no. 5 (December 1986): 1053, https://doi.org/10.2307/1864376.

JULIE A. FAIRMAN
School of Nursing University of Pennsylvania
Philadelphia, PA 19104

The Historian and the Activist: How to Tell Stories that Matter

WENDY KLINE

Purdue University

"A reminder of what to worry about," Susan Reverby wrote on her Facebook page on New Year's day, 2018, returning home to discover that severe weather left her without Internet, phone, or cable. "Call Comcast: guy is coming. Get to the office and discover left half the computer plug at the Cape. Get in the car, drive to Apple Store, buy replacement plug, go back to the office. All annoying, all fixable." These are life's distractions, often keeping us from writing, doing, or seeing what we need to. "The other things:" she continued, "commitment to more resistance, fight for solidarity worldwide, more work, not so easy a fix, but the real things to worry about." Wise words from a woman who has spent her career committed to resistance and solidarity.

Since the beginning of her career, Reverby has sought to balance these challenges—the mundane yet fixable tasks—along with those too overwhelming to always confront. In the early 1970s, Reverby, who self-identified as a "leftist feminist critic of the healthcare system" channeled her activism through the Health Policy Advisory Center in New York City. She sought solutions to healthcare problems (affordability, accessibility, decision making, power, community-based decision-making, prevention, representation, etc.). She also aimed to empower and educate groups of women with the Health/PAC "rap," as it was called.

But she was confounded by the response. No matter what she said, the types of questions she would get were "bipolar in distribution."[1] Half would be far too broad to result in practical change (how to take on US capitalism); the other half far too narrow (how to treat vaginal itch). At the time, she viewed this as a real problem. "The activist in me was often stymied by this repeated experience and stumbling to figure out how these divisions could be reconciled," she reflected. Three decades later, she perceived it differently. "The historian in me thinks that this problem was not so much a division as a

Nursing History Review 27 (2019): 99–103. A Publication of the American Association for the History of Nursing. Copyright © 2019 Springer Publishing Company.
http://dx.doi.org/10.1891/1062-8061.27.99

tension, a tension that all of us trying to think about health policy and feminism will have to consider."[2]

These reflections resulted in an essay, "Thinking through the Body and the Body Politic: Feminism, History, and Health-Care Policy in the United States," a call to arms that was a source of inspiration to me (and to many others) to rethink the history of women's health activism. But it also, more generally, takes historians to task for how we tell our stories. "We tell complicated stories about the past," she explains, but "the result is that those who make policy ... tend to ignore us." They create the histories they want, "finding safety in uncomplicated historical narratives."[3]

Is it possible to be both a good historian and a good activist? The past is complicated. Reverby knows this firsthand; in part because of the fact that the historian in her and the activist in her are lived experiences. Being both historian and activist helped her recognize that what she initially interpreted as a problem also contained a solution.

Reverby uses the recent history of the women's health movement to illustrate what she means in this essay, but her point could be applied to other stories and histories as well. "I worry that we have been very bad historians of our own lifetimes," she admits. Why did her students demonstrate more familiarity with the 19th-century water cure than 1970s feminist politics? What was lost in the telling of personal stories? Because surely there were plenty of stories, and a growing number of voices, who recognized that individual stories mattered.

But how do you tell the stories, and what do you do with them? Part of the complication stemmed from the feminist assumption that the only thing holding women back in the 1970s was knowledge. The acquisition of knowledge would lead to power, as the saying goes. "We thought that with more knowledge and information we were in our own ways making and demanding new policies," writes Reverby.[4] But knowledge was not enough to combat the challenges that divided women, such as racism or classism or homophobia. And these issues prevented women's health activists from creating a united front. Instead, there were multiple strategies, complex coalitions, and lots of tension. The results are still with us today.

The challenge for historians is to understand and interpret these multiple stories. "It would be convenient in telling these stories if these differing strategies would fall neatly into historical periods we could wall off with dates and major events," Reverby explains. "But the reality is that they will not."[5] Intensely personal experiences involving everything from childbirth to racism to rape affected how individuals and groups positioned themselves within the movement. How, then can we write about the recent past which allows for the diversity of experience, the shifting concerns and strategies that shaped women's health in the late 20th century? And further, how can we get policymakers to listen to our stories?

Reverby then turned to her own revelation to suggest a strategy. Remember that initially she perceived the healthcare questions she received as problematic. They were either too insular or too broad and thus could not lead to effective changes. Yet upon historical reflection, she reframed the issue as a tension, rather than a problem. Rather than ignore the tension, she suggests we should embrace it. "We can use the tension between the body and the body politic . . . to examine the kinds of demands women have made and how they have made them." In other words, to do justice to the women's health movement, we need to engage with that tension, rather than to wish it away.

It takes a talented, courageous, and motivated scholar to do this effectively, in such a way that doesn't mask the complications of the past and yet still tells a good story. With the publication of *Examining Tuskegee*, Reverby proved herself up to the task. The Tuskegee study, she argues, has become "both invisible and hypervisible."[6] The way the story has been told and retold, memorialized, and embellished upon requires an acknowledgement of the "messiness of both past and present" and why it is "often ignored and never fully capable of articulation."[7] Reverby's analysis is refreshing in part because it refuses to provide a simple storyline. Exploring contradictions and complexities can yield even better narratives. And if done effectively, even policymakers may pay attention.

Reverby's mission appears more vital than ever before, as the Trump presidency and the #MeToo movement have propelled American women into action. The 2017 Women's March on Washington was likely, according to a *Washington Post* report, the "largest single-day demonstration in recorded U.S. history."[8] Not surprisingly, Reverby was among the marchers. In a recently televised panel discussion, she recalled how different the 2017 march felt to her from other events, such as when she marched in protest against the nomination of Clarence Thomas for the Supreme Court. "I had this feeling that all of us who would be there would try to voice a sense of the country in a much different way," she said of the 2017 march. "I really want to be in the belly of the beast and I want to be there and sort of express my outrage that he was elected and to be part of a group of people who were going to say not just today but every day since you've been elected, we will do something about this."[9] She may have retired from teaching history, but activist Reverby continues the fight.

Have we as historians succeeded in creating uncomplicated stories about the past? Are policymakers listening? Trump and #MeToo have forced us to rethink where we are today and how we possibly got here. Many of us who thought of ourselves more as historians than activists have discovered that the only way to move forward is to embrace activism; to insist that history matters, and to make our voices heard.

So, for example, When the *Washington Post* broke the story in December 2017 that the Trump administration was planning to prohibit the Centers for Disease Control and Prevention from using particular words and phrases in official documents—including the word "fetus"—I pounced. My OpEd, "Trump's Latest Assault on Women: Why Banning the CDC from Using Certain Words has Major Political Ramifications," was published by the *Washington Post* three days later.[10] What was clear to me (and inspired by Susan Reverby) was that such a battle over words, particularly those linked to reproduction, has been part of the longer historical struggle to reclaim knowledge of and power over our bodies. Efforts to ban words such as "fetus" attack the agenda of women's health activists, who have challenged the language surrounding these issues to increase women's control over their own bodies. Since the 1970s, feminists have used the power of the written word to demand bodily rights—birth control, abortion, freedom from coercive sterilization, choices in childbirth—as part of their quest to achieve full equality. The banned words don't just try to silence women, they attempt to dismantle these feminist gains. This may appear obvious to us academics, but many *Washington Post* readers were not familiar with this history.

Back in 2003, when Reverby published her essay "Thinking through the Body," she worried about the fact that students seemed to have so little knowledge the activist contributions of her generation. For my generation, I worried about the fact that so few of my students had even heard of Anita Hill. At least now those voices and stories are getting heard. Young women are listening, and we historians are learning to speak out, to help guide these voices, or at least to provide them with a platform so that they realize that speaking truth to power is not just a current trend; it's the cultivation of generations of struggle.

Reverby continues to remind us of the ways in which 1970s feminist activism prepared us for today. Awed by what she saw at the 2017 women's march, she sensed the myriad personal reasons that brought marchers together, along with the larger political movement that was building. And while it was different than previous protests, she could see the connection to 1970s feminism. "So it's almost like—you should excuse the expression—being back in a consciousness-raising group and that sense of everybody speaks their truth in this time and then they're speaking their truth to power very clearly," she remarked in a panel discussion. "I thought that was great."[11]

Susan Reverby has inspired many scholars and students, academics, and activists. Her teaching, her writing, and her passion to enact change and challenge the status quo serve as a great example of how activism and research can go hand in hand. Engaging in one does not compromise the other; if anything, it can enhance and enrich our understanding of the past and our dreams for the future.

Notes

1.   Reverby, "Thinking through the Body and the Body Politic: Feminism, History, and Health-Care Policy in the United States," in Feldberg, Ladd-Taylor, Li, and McPherson, eds., *Women, Health, and Nation: Canada and the United States* since (1945) (McGill-Queens University Press, 2003), p. 409.

2.   Ibid.

3.   Ibid., 406.

4.   Ibid., 411.

5.   Ibid., 414.

6.   Susan Reverby, *Examining Tuskegee: The Infamous Syphilis Study and Its Legacy* (UNC Press, 2013), p. 6.

7.   Ibid.

8.   This is what we learned by counting the women's marches. https://www.washingtonpost.com/news/monkey-cage/wp/2017/02/07/this-is-what-we-learned-by-counting-the-womens-marches/?utm_term=.126abd7a2efb, viewed (January 9, 2018).

9.   Cambridge Community Television https://www.cctvcambridge.org/wewhomarch.

10.   Trump's latest assault on women https://www.washingtonpost.com/news/made-by-history/wp/2017/12/18/trumps-latest-assault-on-women/?utm_term=.7a18d813b709.

11.   https://www.cctvcambridge.org/wewhomarch, viewed (January 9, 2018).

Wendy Kline, PhD
Department of History
Purdue University

NOTES AND DOCUMENTS

Nursing Diploma to University Education: A Memoir

ELLEN D. BAER
University of Pennsylvania

Last year (2017) marked my 55th reunion with classmates from my undergraduate nursing program, now called Columbia University School of Nursing. In my day, it was still the Columbia University-Presbyterian Hospital School of Nursing. The reunion sparked recollections, ruminations, and insights that begged to be analyzed and spoken. This essay presents my thoughts, spoken first in a presentation at Columbia's reunion.

My undergraduate program was, essentially, a hospital diploma nursing program that built on 2 years of liberal arts college work taken elsewhere. On entry to nursing, I transferred out of my previous 4-year college, after completing 2 years, into the existing 3-year diploma program that had been founded in 1892 as the Presbyterian Hospital School of Nursing. It was a marvelous program at top ranked Columbia Presbyterian Medical Center in New York City. We all became clinical experts in our 3 years working 28-hour weeks staffing the medical center in every imaginable specialty area, at all shifts, four seasons a year, added to classes taught by very well-known Medical Center physicians and nurses, and only 4 weeks of vacation every summer. At graduation, we received a nursing diploma from Presbyterian Hospital and a Bachelor of Science from Columbia.

Today, that program is a fully accredited graduate school at Columbia University, offering highly regarded masters and doctorates for nurse practitioners, nurse midwives, nurse anesthetists, nurse researchers, and health policy experts. Some beginning nurses still attend the school, but they all have

Nursing History Review 27 (2019): 104–109. A Publication of the American Association for the History of Nursing. Copyright © 2019 Springer Publishing Company.
http://dx.doi.org/10.1891/1062-8061.27.104

obtained baccalaureates in other fields and enter as second-degree students into the nursing major, enroute to their graduate degrees; it's called Masters Direct Entry. The school has become a graduate school, in keeping with all of Columbia's other professional schools. The faculty run and practice nursing at a successful, independent nurse practitioner clinical practice facility. How did this evolution occur?

We all know how the story began.

I like to talk about history using concepts to describe the essence of history; that history is made when the right people meet in the right place at the right time.

And so it is consistent with history that nursing happened in times of war, when an upper class educated British woman, Florence Nightingale, went to the Crimea to help care for British soldiers, at a time when the British empire was at its full power; and an important British war correspondent, Sidney Herbert, wrote about what Nightingale did in British newspapers. The British public showered monetary gifts on her that she used to open and endow a nursing school, St Thomas in London. And, because of Britain's importance in that time, word spread around the British Empire, even to its former colony, the United States.

Notable Americans like Louisa Mae Alcott, Clara Barton, and Walt Whitman went into American Civil War battlefields to care for the wounded, and wrote about it. And after that war, committees founded during the war, with members from the upper classes, took an interest in other people displaced by social upheaval and formed Visiting Committees to visit social establishments like hospitals, almshouses, and prisons, to see how the inhabitants fared, and they wrote about it.

One such visitor at Bellevue told a compelling tale. As she visited, the wards to see how people were managing in the city almshouses and early hospitals, Elizabeth Hobson found:

> When the visitor entered the ward the [untrained] nurse was absent in the operating room where a woman was in operation for cancer – a little boy of 5 years old had just been operated upon for stones in the bladder, an old woman [a patient] was sitting by him trying good naturedly to soothe his cries but doing nothing to staunch the blood which was flowing from the wound.[1]

In other words, kindness was not enough. Caretaking required knowledge.

Hobson and her fellow social reformers, all society women, sought to solve the problem by following Nightingale's model, creating the New York Training School for Nurses at Bellevue in 1873. The New York reformers raised the funds and started the school over the objections of many physicians and clergymen who opposed the entry of women into such laborious work with often disreputable patients.

Why schools? In the 1800s, it was not considered proper for women to work outside of their homes, and the social reformers who created nursing wanted their nurses to be proper young women. So, they called the facilities schools and placed a matron in charge to manage discipline and teach what little technique was then known.

After Bellevue's founding came the Connecticut Training School (later Yale), the Boston Training School (later Massachusetts General Hospital), and the New York Hospital Training School (later Cornell). As recognition of the efficiency and efficacy of nursing grew, hospitals all over the country adopted the plan. By 1880, there were 15 schools; by 1900, 432 schools.[2]

My school is one of the few schools of nursing that has maintained its existence through almost the entire history of modern, trained nursing. It evolved from a hospital diploma school founded in 1892 to its current University degree granting enterprise, without interruption of services, and only a few bumps along the way.

Please realize that, as the pupil nurses at the hospital schools provided all of the patient care in the related hospitals, the graduates of the schools were not hired to staff the hospitals. Instead they went into private duty nursing in people's homes. Visiting nursing and other public health practices emerged as well, that employed some of the graduate nurses.

But work for the graduate nurses was sporadic and disorganized. As a result, in the 1890s, the Training School Directors formed associations such as the Superintendents Society (later the NLN) and the Associated Alumnae Association (later the ANA). The Superintendents Society focused on streamlining curricula and setting school standards. The ANA set up nurses' registries to organize graduate nurses available for private duty, so that families could seek help in a central location. The Alumna associations also arranged benefits for nurses who became ill and could no longer work for pay.

Remember, this time preceded social security, workers' compensation, and other supports for people who grew too old, sick, or disabled to work; including single women such as nurses who had no families to support them in their declining years. And in those years most nurses were required to be single women.

Historical events continued to impact nursing throughout the history of my school. Just think of the 1900s: World War I occurred in the 19s; followed by the depression which lasted from 1929 until the late 1930s and had a grave impact on graduate nurses because families that lost their money in the depression could no longer afford to hire private nurses to care for their sick family members.

Terrible economic conditions for graduate nurses caused politicians, social agents, and nurses to press hospitals to begin to employ graduate nurses, which slowly, they did.[3]

Then World War II (WWII) occurred in the early 1940s, during which many new medical advances were utilized on the battle fields. Among them were anesthesia, blood transfusion, and penicillin for infected wounds. Adapting such battle field practices to domestic hospitals called for additional education for nurses. Happily, WWII also led to the GI Bill, which provided economic support to members of the armed services to go to college, including nurses.[4]

As nurses earned baccalaureate and advanced degrees, they were able to attain higher ranks in hospitals, industry, research, and universities. Having nurses at higher levels provided opportunities for them to include other nurses and promote nurses abilities to contribute at higher levels of society.

But more challenging eras were coming for nursing.

One historian of health care, Nancy Tomes, wrote an article about nursing entitled "A Little World of Our Own."[5] The title is so revealing because I do think nurses view nursing's place in the world from within nursing, rather than as part of an entire historical era. Nursing has suffered from that view.

Alumni, such as my colleagues at Columbia, have blamed their schools for events over which the schools had little control. During the 1960s, era of social protests about civil rights and women's rights, is it really any surprise that nursing enrollments declined? That women sought entry to other professions previously denied to them? Was that the fault of nursing? Of course not. From the other side, the schools (such as mine) blamed alumni for not coming to the support of the schools as they lost status because of declining enrollments and imperiled finances. As nursing school enrollments declined at Columbia, nursing buildings were taken over for other uses, as dorms for other students and offices for members of other professions. The unkindest cut of all was the destruction of Columbia Presbyterian nursing's main dorm and classroom building, Maxwell Hall, to allow for the construction of a new hospital on its site, the Milstein Hospital, a core building of what has become New York-Presbyterian Hospital/Columbia Medical Center. To this day, many of us cannot enter that hospital building without feeling the loss.

In toto, a sea change occurred in the identity of Columbia nursing in those years. For close to 100 years, the school's foci and identity had resided within the old nursing school building and the old hospitals, which we knew like the backs of our hands. With new hospital buildings, and no more nursing dorms, the identity of nursing education shifted to the University, with which we had almost no relationship.

But the ebbs and flows of history work in the other direction as well. Nursing has emerged from that era in better condition: nurses are better educated, more autonomous, and gain better recognition for their contributions. The reason for that, again, is history.

By 1965 Congress had created Medicare and Medicaid that produced enormous numbers of newly insured citizens seeking general wellness and geriatric care. There were not enough physicians to provide that care, which led to the development of Nurse Practitioner programs all over the United States.[6] My old school has been one of the leaders in developing such programs. And just this spring, Columbia dedicated its brand-new state of the art School of Nursing building on its Medical Center campus at 168th Street.

Now nurses are earning masters' and doctoral degrees and taking their places in board rooms and senate hearings and the National Institutes of Health, where the momentous decisions that affect health care are being made. In 2010, the Institute of Medicine issued a strong report, "The Future of Nursing," calling for 80% of all nurses to be prepared at the baccalaureate or higher degree level by 2020 to keep pace with the rising demands of huge areas of knowledge in patient care. One cannot help but believe that the presence of nurse members within the Institute of Medicine made that statement possible. And those nurse members are all part of nursing's new highly educated professorial cohort.

I confess that I mourn for that lost era of nursing in its own little world. It was an extended family; a source of great accomplishment and pride; a place where I became a confident, competent, serious adult woman. But I have also been fortunate to have found a new world in university nursing, also like family and marked by wonderful group accomplishments and success. So, I have concluded that, in evolving, we all experience loss, but hopefully find new growth and achievement that makes our present and future rich and rewarding.

Notes

1. Elizabeth C. Hobson, *Recollections of a Happy Life* (New York: G. P. Putnam's Sons, 1916). See also, "Report of the Chairman of Surgical Wards for Women," November 22, 1872. New York: Frederick L. Ehrman Medical Library, NYU School of Medicine, 1872.

2. Lavinia L. Dock, *A History of Nursing*, Volume III (New York: G. P. Putnam's Sons, 1912), p. 141.

3. Jean C. Whelan, "'A Necessity in the Nursing World': The Chicago Nurses Professional Registry, 1913–1950." *Nursing History Review*, 2005; 13:49–75.

4. Ellen D. Baer, "'A Cooperative Venture': In Search of Professional Status: A Research Journal for Nursing," *Nursing Research*, 1987; 36: 18–25.

5. Nancy Tomes, "Little World of our Own: The Pennsylvania Hospital Training School for Nurses, 1895–1907," *Journal of the History of Medicine and Allied Science*, 1978; 33:507–530.

6. Ellen D. Baer, "A Philosophical Argument Supporting Primary Care Nursing." In Mezey, M. & McGivern, D. *Nurses, Nurse Practitioners: The Evolution of Primary Care* (Boston, MA: Little, Brown, 1986), 15–28.

ELLEN D. BAER, RN, PhD, FAAN
Professor Emerita of Nursing
University of Pennsylvania
Philadelphia, PA 19104

IN MEMORIAM

Louise Fitzpatrick, EdD, RN, FAAN: March 24, 1942–September 1, 2017

Dean Louise Fitzpatrick, a towering figure in both the nursing education and the history of nursing, died on September 1, 2017 after a 3-year struggle with cancer. Many will remember Dean Fitzpatrick for her steadfast commitment to nursing as a force that can better the lives of individuals and families at home and around the globe. Many will also her commitment to the highest standards of nursing education, one expressed in her success in securing Villanova University's College of Nursing's repeated designation as a Center of Excellence by the National League for Nursing. Villanova's alumni and supporters will remember her steadfast support of its basketball Wildcats through all of the years of her deanship.

I will remember someone who, quite honestly, scared me to death when I first met her. As a first semester, first-year doctoral student I met Dean Fitzpatrick at a history of health care conference at the Pennsylvania Hospital in the fall of 1984. I needed no introduction to her: I knew her work so well. I had read *The National Organization for Public Health Nursing 1912–1952* (New York: National League for Nursing, 1975); *Prologue to Professionalism: A History of Nursing* (Bowie, MD: R.J. Brady, 1983); and *Nursing in Society: A Historical Perspective* (Philadelphia: W.B. Saunders, 1983). Little did I know that Dean Fitzpatrick was also beginning her service on the Advisory Board of what would become the Barbara Bates Center for the Study of the History of Nursing, then only a vision held by Joan Lynaugh, Karen Buhler-Wilkerson and Ellen Baer.

Of course, I very quickly came to know Dean Fitzpatrick as a wise and wonderful advisor, scholar, and champion of nursing and nursing history. I came to know her as a proud native of South River, New Jersey. I learned of her education at the Johns Hopkins School of Nursing, where she focused her work on public health in the city of Baltimore. Dean Fitzpatrick went on to earn a BSN from the Catholic University of America, and her MA, Med, and EdD from Columbia University.

Nursing History Review 27 (2019): 110–111. A Publication of the American Association for the History of Nursing. Copyright © 2019 Springer Publishing Company.
http://dx.doi.org/10.1891/1062-8061.27.110

Dean Fitzpatrick's many honors included the Distinguished Alumni Award of the Johns Hopkins Alumni Association; the National League for Nursing's Award for Outstanding Leadership in Nursing Education; an honorary degree from Villanova; the Nurse as Global Citizen Award of the Pennsylvania State Nurses Association; and the Legion of Honor Gold Medallion of the Four Chaplains Memorial Foundation. She was also Fellow of the American Academy of Nursing and served as President of the Pennsylvania Higher Education Nursing Schools Association.

On September 6, 2017, Villanova University memorialized Dean Fitzpatrick's life and the many illustrious contributions she made to her community, her discipline, her University, and her world with a Mass of Christian Burial at St. Thomas' Church. She was buried on September 7, at the Holy Cross Cemetery and Mausoleum near her hometown in Jamesburg, New Jersey. Villanova has established the Dean M. Louise Fitzpatrick Fund, which honors her memory. Contributions may be made to the Fund at Villanova University College of Nursing, 800 E. Lancaster Avenue, Villanova, PA 19085.

An early version of this remembrance of Dean Fitzpatrick appeared in *The Chronicle* of the Barbara Bates Center for the Study of the History of Nursing.

Patricia D'Antonio, PhD, RN, FAAN
Carol E. Ware Professor of Psychiatric Mental Health Nursing
University of Pennsylvania School of Nursing

MEDIA REVIEWS

Mercy Street: A Six-part Civil War Drama. 2016. PBS, Executive Producer: Ridley Scott; Directors: Rex Ann Dawson and Jeremy Welsh (360 minutes on 2 discs)

Heroines of Mercy Street: The Real Nurses of the Civil War, by Pamela D. Toler. 2016. New York: Back Bay Books, Little, Brown and Company, 287 pages; $16.99

Based on the original diary and letters of Mary Phinney von Olnhausen, a widow who served at Mansion House Hospital in Alexandria, Virginia, in 1862, the television series *Mercy Street* captures the essence of the struggles volunteer nurses faced during the American Civil War.[1] The series is set in Mansion House Hospital, a hotel confiscated by the Union for use as a hospital in the Union occupied town on the outskirts of Washington, DC (it is now a museum and open for tours). It is here that Phinney, a staunch New England abolitionist, is sent to work by Dorothea Dix, superintendent of nursing for the Union. And it is at Mansion House, renamed "Mercy Street Hospital" for the fictional series, that Phinney collides with military surgeons who do not want meddling women volunteers interfering in their military system. She also encounters Anne Hastings (a character based on the historical figure Anne Reading, a British nurse), and Miss Emma Green (a young southern belle whose family owns the hotel, and whose loyalties lie with the Confederacy).

From my knowledge of nursing history during the Civil War, the conflicts between nurse Phinney and the Union surgeons are accurately portrayed in the series. In addition, the show accurately documents the inefficiencies and corruption in the system, particularly related to the misuse and misdirection of supplies, foods, and medicines meant for the soldiers. Other aspects, including the depiction of rampant disease in crowded, makeshift hospitals; the shortage of nurses; and the overworked and often-unskilled physicians; the lack of private rooms for nurses; and the conflicts between the surgeons and Miss Dix (sometimes referred to as "Dragon Dix"), are also correct. From a theatrical perspective, the costumes and dialogue are appropriate to the era, and the narrative tension and pace of the series holds ones'

Nursing History Review 27 (2019): 112–114. A Publication of the American Association for the History of Nursing. Copyright © 2019 Springer Publishing Company.
http://dx.doi.org/10.1891/1062-8061.27.112

interest. On the other hand, aspects of the series are melodramatic—such as that of the dying young soldier whose hand is glued with dried blood to the US flag.

Of particular interest is the depiction of the British nurse who claimed to have worked with Florence Nightingale in the Crimea. Phinney references such a nurse in her original diary, *Adventures of an Army Nurse* (1904), and describes their run-ins at Mansion House Hospital, as well as Anne Hasting's drinking problem. According to the producer, the series drew material for those scenes from the diary of Anne Reading, a nurse who worked in the Crimea for a few months and then traveled to the United States in the late 1850s.[2] Dramatically portrayed in the series, nonetheless, the character embodied traits typical of some pre-professional nurses of the era.

Taking the viewer beyond the hospital scenes, the television series also addresses the problems of freed and runaway slaves, the corruption in the military, and the extent to which the Green family members will go to preserve their way of life and demonstrate their loyalty to the Confederacy. All of these provide additional context in a show that uses the lens of social history to make its case.

In contrast to the television series, the book *Heroines of Mercy Street* is a factual history written with a social history framework. In it, author Pamela Todler takes the reader beyond Alexandria, Virginia, and provides a brief overview of the highlights of nursing and medicine in the Civil War, relying on numerous secondary sources to do so. The exception to the use of secondary sources is the chapter on Mary Phinney that is based on her diary and letters (compiled in 1904). In this chapter, Todler provides a precise and accurate account of Phinney's work in the war, both in Alexandria and in Moorehead City, North Carolina in 1863. The descriptive narrative, engaging in tone and accurate in its facts, is an easy read—one that both the general public and the nursing community would enjoy.

Both the book and the *Mercy Street* television series would be of interest to anyone seeking a brief overview of nursing in the pre-professional era of the American Civil War, 1861–1865, although neither are scholarly historical critiques. The television series is particularly useful in the classroom. I have used excerpts from *Mercy Street* in class to engage students and initiate discussion comparing the original Phinney diary (primary source) to the video and found the students' reactions to be very positive. Some scenes can lay the groundwork for engaging students in a discussion of the ethical dilemmas nurses and physicians faced during the war, particularly the notion of neutrality on the part of health care providers. Addressing that ethical dilemma is in fact the major premise of the show: as is stated on the cover-case "blood is neither gray nor blue."[3] Additionally, the series provides an ideal context for discussions of the effects of race, class, and gender on women's work in the mid-19th century.

Notes

1. Mary Phinney von Olnhausen, *Adventures of an Army Nurse in Two Wars* (Boston, MA: Little Brown, 1904).
2. Ridley Scott, in Pamela Todler, *Heroines of Mercy Street* (2016): Foreword viii.
3. Ridley Scott, *Mercy Street: A Six-part Civil War Drama* (PBS: 2016).

ARLENE W. KEELING, PhD, RN, FAAN
Professor Emerita
School of Nursing
The University of Virginia
Claude Moore Nursing Education Building
225 Jeanette Lancaster Way
Charlottesville, VA 22908

Celebrating History: Health Informatics at 50. Author: Dominique Tobbell Academic Health Center, Institute for Health Informatics, University of Minnesota. https://healthinformatics.umn.edu/history

Celebrating History: Health Informatics at 50 fetes the University of Minnesota's (UMN) Institute for Health Informatics at its 50th Anniversary. The website highlights the program's history, milestones, and its pioneering members through text, images, an interactive timeline, and 10 oral histories. Housed within the Institute's website, the "History" section provides an overview of health informatics at UMN. It traces the Institute's origins to 1965 when the National Institutes of Health awarded a grant to establish a Biomedical Data Processing Unit. The site describes the expansion of the program, including graduate education and new initiatives in biomedical computing.

The main History page provides an overview of the Institute's achievements and features an interactive timeline at the bottom of the page. Users can scroll through events along the timeline beginning with the 1962 establishment of a committee to investigate forming a biomedical computing facility within the College of Medical Sciences. Events in the timeline are categorized in three "streams": Firsts, Innovations, and Milestones. Each item on the timeline is marked with a brief note of its historical significance. Clicking on that timeline item brings viewers to the expanded description in the window above. Viewers can also page through the expanded descriptions chronologically to view images of faculty and descriptions of key moments in the Institutes' history, with the timeline below marking the viewers' progress through the content.

Scholars interested in the history of health informatics can find a potential treasure trove of information as they navigate through the three other pages on the site. Two short articles on particular elements of the Institute's history establish the unique nature of health informatics research and practice developed at UMN. The first: "Fifty Years of Health Informatics Innovation" page provides an overview of the most salient features of UMN's program. The page discusses a range of innovations developed at the University, including: population-based models of epidemic simulations; telehealth and at-home monitoring for cystic fibrosis; clinical decision-making tools; and the development of a database that "contains information on microbial biocatalytic reactions and biodegradation pathways for primarily xenobiotic, chemical compounds." The second article: "A 50-Year Commitment to Interprofessionalism" chronicles the Institute's long practice of working across disciplines.

Nursing History Review 27 (2019): 115–117. A Publication of the American Association for the History of Nursing. Copyright © 2019 Springer Publishing Company.
http://dx.doi.org/10.1891/1062-8061.27.115

Beginning in the 1960s with cardiologists, pediatricians, and epidemiologists the institute rapidly expanded beyond medical specialties, becoming a center of study for nursing informatics in the 1980s, and adding dental and veterinary practitioners in the 1990s.

Dominique Tobbell, a UMN faculty member and historian of 20th-century health care, biomedical science, and technology, authored the site and its two articles. She ties each of the innovations to the faculty member who developed them, including many of the Institute's founding members.

The interviews Dr. Tobbell conducted are found on the "Oral History Project" page, which provides brief biographies of 10 faculty members. Each interviewee has their own page that includes a biographical sketch, interview abstract, and a link to the interview transcript. The transcripts range in length from 7 to 32 pages, with most being approximately 25 pages.

The "Oral History Project" and transcripts offer a rich source for historians and medical professionals interested in health informatics. Dr. Tobbell not only deftly traces the innovations of each faculty member, she also engages them in conversations that consider the culture of the Institute, how that changed over time, and the ways in which faculty collaborated with one another. That so many of the interviews discuss collaboration with female faculty and researchers is striking, especially in contrast to the demographics of the timeline, and the presence of only one woman in the oral history interviews. Yet, the role of women and gender is an interesting theme that runs throughout conversations. The interviews also provide nuanced dimensions to the history of informatics at UMN, including the personal and interpersonal factors that structured the program such as spousal hires, cross-country moves, and the origins of collaborative projects. These details are often lost in institutional histories, yet they highlight the importance of personal connections.

"Celebrating History: Health Informatics at 50" has many strengths and benefits, particularly for professionals with an interest in, and knowledge of, health informatics. Those less familiar with the field may find it difficult to decipher the field-specific terminology. Others may find women under-represented, particularly given the references to their presence in the oral histories, and the importance of the nursing informatics research conducted at the Institute. However, more may be forthcoming, as transcripts indicate that Dr. Tobbell completed interviews not yet available through the site. Finally, the project was completed as part of the 50th Anniversary of the Institute for Health Informatics, and as such is focused on the specific contributions of UMN faculty. As a result, it understandably provides less historical context and framing than a broader history of health informatics would.

The strengths of the site far outweigh the shortcomings. The content provides a great source of data and information regarding the history of a field that continues to shape health care today. With the current health care climate that is often consumed with discussions of health informatics, its benefits and potential drawbacks, this website provides an intriguing glimpse into to the origins of the field within a specific institutional setting.

MEGHAN CRNIC, PhD
Lecturer, Undergraduate Research Coordinator
History and Sociology of Science
University of Pennsylvania
249 S. 36th Street, 303 Cohen Hall
Philadelphia, PA 19104

REVIEW ESSAY

Mrs. Stone & Dr. Smellie: Eighteenth-Century Midwives and their Patients
By Robert Woods and Chris Galley (Liverpool, UK: Liverpool University Press, 2014) (544 pages; $110 cloth)

The Birth of Mankind: Otherwise Named, The Woman's Book
Edited by Elaine Hobby (New York, NY; Routledge Taywlor and Francis Group, 2009) (310 pages; $150 cloth, $56.00 e-book)

These books represent both popular and scientific writing about the management of birth from the 16th to the 18th centuries. Although originally published nearly 200 years apart, they are unified in an attempt to manage common maladies of pregnancy and infancy, a period of particular vulnerability for women even today. *The Birth of Mankind* is a manual of care for pregnant women and infants, with additional information on basic anatomy and remedies for common health complaints, published in Britain in 1540, with many subsequent editions remaining in publication until 1654. Aimed at a general rather than a medical audience, the text provides recipes and guidelines for management of various birth and medical situations. *Mrs. Stone & Dr. Smellie*, on the other hand, is a collection of case notes by consultant midwives practicing in England between 1700s and 1750s. Their published cases are instructional lessons for other midwifery practitioners, detailing difficult cases and the appropriate management to preserve the lives of both baby and mother, or at least the mother in the worst situations. Each of these texts provides rich detail on the practice of midwifery, and medicine more generally, over more than a century, and the incidental details they shed on life, health, and care will interest scholars from many different fields.

Hobby's introduction to *The Birth of Mankind* puts the book in the context of its period. She makes special note of its publishing history as she details the transfer of copyright from one author/publisher to the next, over a century. In doing so, she identifies textual changes to correct blatant errors or misinformation that were removed or corrected. Hobby notes that although the book was widely distributed throughout the 16th century, it has been

Nursing History Review 27 (2019): 118–121. A Publication of the American Association for the History of Nursing. Copyright © 2019 Springer Publishing Company.
http://dx.doi.org/10.1891/1062-8061.27.118

overlooked in studies of British life in that era, with no modern editions issued for scholars, an omission that Hobby sought to remedy.

The Birth of Mankind was a translation from an earlier German midwifery textbook, where midwives studied and then had an examination on their practice. Due to the less stringent regulation of midwifery in Britain, the English translation of this text was aimed at a more general audience, and initially contained many erroneous treatments. The text was divided into four books. Beginning in Book 1 with a detailed explanation of the anatomy of the reproductive organs and breasts, Book 2 focuses on birth, both normal and with complications. Book 3 covers care of the infant and Book 4 involves conception and methods to treat infertility. Original illustrations are featured in Books 1 and 2 to supplement the text.

Hobby provides extensive annotations to support the reader. The book includes a glossary, but most useful are the footnotes within the text that offer the reader immediate translation for unfamiliar terms or phrases. While some terms may be relatively clear (privy parts for private parts, for instance), others are more difficult to understand, such as matrix for womb or reaching for clearing the throat. Hobby also identifies where text changed over the course of various editions, noting the source of new material, and information about content that was removed. A modern reader will recognize the illustrations, many of which were originally copied from earlier well-known texts. For readers familiar with labor and birth many of the complaints or birth circumstances are familiar. Methods for easing and provoking labor occupy a large portion of Book 2, as do instructions for managing difficult fetal presentations. Treatments recommended for laboring women include enemas to induce labor or to provide nutrition, and soporifics to induce sleep for exhausted laboring women. Some of these were likely quite helpful, while others offered little benefit. Most likely any of the methods, when used by an experienced midwife would be more successful than a random or poorly timed application of treatments by a less-practiced midwife. The next text is an effort to define those appropriate techniques and applications.

Woods and Galley's *Mrs. Stone & Dr. Smellie* is a presentation of two consultant midwives' case histories of midwifery care in the 1700s. As consultant midwives *Mrs. Stone & Dr. Smellie* were both in the position of being called to attend to births after the first (or second) midwife failed to achieve a birth. Both midwives published their case studies as an effort to improve the care of laboring women by improving midwifery practice overall. The book is made up of multiple chapters that can stand alone, or be read as presented. Beginning with an overview of midwifery in England in the 18th century, the authors put Stone's and Smellie's published cases in the context of midwifery care in the era, as well as within the context of medical publications. The authors further dedicate their second chapter to the nuances of reading published case notes.

The authors provide chapter-length biographies of both Stone and Smellie, and offer historic and demographic analysis of the midwives' cases in the chapter preceding the respective case notes. Mrs. Stone's *Complete Practice* is reproduced in full, with all 43 cases included. A collection of 22 of Smellie's cases are reproduced, focusing on the years of his London practice, and grouped by topic. Stone and Smellie describe similar births and complications, but they use different language—Stone using more colloquial descriptions, while Smellie uses more technical language. Interestingly, however, both encourage their readers to foster good relations with other midwives, and to act with care to prevent injury to the mother or baby. Woods and Galley are historical demographers, which gives their analytic essays an interesting focus on the actual numbers of births attended, geographic distribution of the practices, and enumeration of maternal and fetal outcomes of the cases. Woods and Galley refer to both practitioners as midwives, recognizing the different path to professional midwifery practice that men and women took in that era. The authors do not weigh in on the debate over man-midwives, rather they note that both men and women practiced concurrently, and often consulting one another when difficult cases arose.

As with Hobby's book, *Mrs. Stone & Dr. Smellie* is thoroughly annotated, offering definitions of unusual terms and providing historical context. Appendices provide supplementary material including a list of anatomy, medical and midwifery textbooks ordered both alphabetically and by year of publication, an essay on the publishing environment for case notes, an essay on prescriptions, and finally a sample of case reports by a contemporary French man-midwife both in French and translated into English.

One of the strengths of *Mrs. Stone & Dr. Smellie* is that it includes well over 100 cases from an extended sample of 23 other midwives. The supplementary cases are from both men and women midwives, all in the latter part of the 18th century. These cases are included in the book as examples of the absence of medical progress in midwifery over the century. The supplementary cases offer different perspectives on the birth process and of midwifery care, but unlike Stone and Smellie, most of the supplementary cases do not provide useful guidance for a practitioner. Rather the supplementary cases publicize the professional experiences of the midwife in question, or serve as a general commentary on midwifery practice. The varieties of management of the persistent problems of malpresentation and hemorrhage are interesting, however, as the supplementary midwives detail their unique approach to each condition. There is a comprehensive summary chapter that precedes the supplementary cases, giving biographical and practice details of each of the midwives featured. Both the summary chapter and the chapter with the cases themselves would benefit from a dedicated table of contents to help the reader more easily find the individual midwives' cases.

For this midwife, the case descriptions were all too familiar. Indeed, I found it hard to tear myself away from the case reports. Being familiar with birth I could understand the physical and intellectual challenges that these 16th- and 18th-century midwives encountered. The majority of difficult cases involved common obstetric emergencies such as malpresentation (breech, shoulder, transverse, or face presentations), pelvic obstruction, and hemorrhage. As a midwife practicing in an acute care setting in the United States, many of these cases are avoided with the availability of ultrasounds and safe cesarean sections. I do not encounter the trauma of an obstructed labor in which a dead fetus must be extracted in pieces to allow the mother to live, although that is still a reality in some places in the world today, and hemorrhage remains a leading cause of maternal mortality around the world.

These books, both foreign and familiar, demonstrate the constancy of some medical problems throughout history. The case notes offer examples of care practices, but also the clinical reasoning used by practitioners. They offer an unusually intimate view into a medical past that could supplement the materials in many different classrooms. Both books can be of interest to historians of midwifery, medicine, and pharmacy, as well as historians of publishing, linguistics, and family life. As reproductions of primary sources, these texts will be useful for scholars unable to travel to the Wellcome library collection to view the originals. Both would make useful additions to university library collections.

WINIFRED C. CONNERTON, PhD, CNM
Assistant Professor
College of Health Professions
Lienhard School of Nursing
Pace University

BOOK REVIEWS

British Women Surgeons and their Patients 1860–1918

By Claire Brock
(Cambridge, UK: Cambridge University Press, 2017)
(305 pages; $92.19 hardcover)

When I agreed to review *British Women Surgeons and their Patients* I had feared a triumphalistic feminist history of women surgeons, but the reality was a much more pragmatic view spanning a fascinating 60-year period between 1860 and 1918. Claire Brock focuses on the changing social and cultural backgrounds to the surgical practices of a number of women and the relationships between them, their male counterparts and their patients.

As well as a well-balanced introduction setting the historical scene from 1860 onwards, and the brief conclusion, it is divided into five main chapters. These take the reader from 1872, at a time when, in the UK, women were fighting to train as doctors, while simultaneously surgeons' professional status was being raised largely due to the introduction of anesthesia and antisepsis. The mid-1860s also saw the rise of an organized campaign for women's rights, later focusing on women's suffrage, so that it is unsurprising to find direct links between these struggles especially in key personalities such as Elizabeth Garrett Anderson.

The first half of the book focuses on the elite women practitioners at the two London hospitals: The New Hospital for Women (NHW) and the Royal Free Hospital (RFH). However, using the word "British" in the title feels rather a misnomer. While there is a brief mention of Sophia Jex-Blake in Edinburgh (p. 17) and of the Birmingham and Midland Hospital for Women, which accepted Louisa Atkins as a house surgeon (pp. 17–18), I felt there was a significant gap here. The 1870s struggle to improve standards of surgery at the NHW fell largely between Garrett Anderson and Atkins. Might a look at the women surgeons employed at the provincial hospitals and the Scottish Hospitals have informed this story and subsequent chapters rather better?

My other criticism is the almost complete lack of any but the briefest of references to nursing throughout the book—"nurse" and "nursing" do not

Nursing History Review 27 (2019): 122–124. A Publication of the American Association for the History of Nursing. Copyright © 2019 Springer Publishing Company.
http://dx.doi.org/10.1891/1062-8061.27.122

even appear in the index—even though the rise of the surgically trained nurse was arguably the third, but often ignored, contributory factor to the rise of effective surgery throughout this period. While we are told how the women surgeons were not able to receive the same form of supervised instruction as students that their male contemporaries received and therefore had to learn "on the job," Brock totally ignores the surgical education of the nursing staff which presumably was part of the surgeons' role?

Despite these remarks, there is much to recommend *British Women Surgeons and their Patients*, not least the wealth of sources upon which Brock has drawn, including the case notes of a large number of patients. The detail in some of these patient narratives is at times fascinating although use of prosopographical data analysis might have added a better analysis of the data. Instead Brock has used a series of abstracts from these to illustrate her points, for example, the repeated dismissal by GPs of symptoms as menopausal, when in fact they should have indicated the presence of malignancy. The sad details these contain are shocking yet reflect well this period of medical and surgical transition and correlation between social inequities and disease. They also illustrate the degree of trepidation demonstrated by patients in what were probably their first forays into a hospital while revealing that the surgeon's gender was of relatively low importance to them.

The final chapter looks at the opportunities opened up to women surgeons in wartime. First within the theater of war, close to the front in non-military as well as military hospitals in France, Greece, and Serbia, and second on the home front as World War I (WWI) resulted in large numbers of male medics signing up, leaving women to fill their places at home often on a locum tenens basis. In Chapter 4, Brock tells a story of initial obstructiveness followed by gradual acceptance and growing professional respect for women surgeons at the front—bearing a striking resemblance to that experienced by women as nurses working with the military in earlier conflicts. The media language also bears a notable similarity, for example, descriptions of the women's "selfless courage" and having "divine fingers" as "ethereal beings" looking benevolently over their charges (pp. 226–229). The site of some of the women's hospitals, a little way from the front, was conducive to experimental treatments in dressings, use of serums and delayed surgery to avoid gas gangrene. The surgeons often found themselves treating the local population with referrals from doctors in the community and Brock emphasizes the hunger with which these women surgeons apparently grasped all and any surgical experiences placed before them.

Likewise, the final chapter covering the experiences of those who either stayed at home or returned home to take up posts, highlights the wealth of opportunities for surgical experience presented to women due to severe difficulties in filling posts normally offered exclusively to men. Students nearing the end of their training acted as assistants and were appointed as house surgeons straight from graduation.

Finishing in 1918 is frustrating in leaving the history at the point at which WWI finished and male surgeons return to their posts—we are left wondering to what extent did the female surgeons have to relinquish their positions and enter a retrograde period? As a fascinating and well-researched book on history of surgery, I strongly recommend this book.

HELEN SWEET, PhD
Research Associate
Wellcome Unit for the History of Medicine, University of Oxford

Psychiatry and Racial Liberalism in Harlem 1836–1968

By Dennis A. Doyle
(University of Rochester Press, Rochester NY, 2017)
(268 pages; $34.95 cloth; $24.99 e-book).

Doyle's comprehensive analysis of attempts to introduce psychiatric services into New York's Harlem communities is the latest book in an emerging body of work, which attempts to address the intersection between race and psychiatry.[1] Doyle's contribution draws on comprehensive archival research to explore the impact of "the psychiatric point of view" on various aspects of health, law, and social control for African Americans living in Central Harlem during the "long civil rights period." The seven main chapters that cover various moments, people, or programs are drawn together by the thematic thread of "racial liberalism," or to what extent did liberals use psychiatry in the context of Civil Rights. Doyle's conclusion is that the language of "liberalism" and attempts at "color blindness" caused as many problems as they sought to solve and failed to deal with any of the structural issues affecting mental health in Harlem in that time period.

Doyle starts his argument with a thorough demonstration of the historically racist nature of American psychiatry. As others have shown, the majority of racial injustice in the United States, including slavery, has been built on the belief that the African American was somehow inherently psychologically inferior, more childlike, or just plain bad.[2] Psychiatry as a rule did little to challenge this belief, and in fact actively contributed to it. It took the effects of the Great Migration on northern white communities before serious attention was paid to the psychology of African American communities but this attention was framed originally in the form of a law and order issue. Doyle details the attempts of New York's Judge Justine Wise Polier and her colleagues to deal with the so-called criminality of black communities by initiating a number of programs informed by the emerging child psychology and child guidance movement. In Chapter 3, Doyle extends this to an analysis of attempts to deal with "juvenile delinquency." This is a complicated term, and there is a tendency at times in the text to use that label unproblematically. In the mid-20th-century social sciences, it was a catch all phrase for young people behaving "badly" but what exactly was the "bad" behavior, and how are we to conceptualize this when it's applied to young African Americans locked into cycles of poverty, oppression, and racist abuse. Doyle tries to unpack these complicated ideas as he explores a number of programs and initiatives designed to intervene in the black community at the level of prevention. These programs were made

Nursing History Review 27 (2019): 125–127. A Publication of the American Association for the History of Nursing. Copyright © 2019 Springer Publishing Company.
http://dx.doi.org/10.1891/1062-8061.27.125

fundable only by linking them to the problem of "crime" rather than overtly addressing individual mental health issues, and the extent to which therapeutic programs based on psychiatric method were actually used is taken up in good critical detail here. That "delinquency" is sometimes conflated with actual criminality (rather than mental illness) in Doyle's text is hardly surprising, given they were not really understood as separate entities at the time—behavior was read as anti-social and a problem for "other" people and so the "problem" of the African American psyche was one of criminality, not really one of trauma or actual serious mental illness. In part, this also reflects the nature of American psychiatry in the pre- and immediate post-war period as concerned more with social stability rather than individual health for its own sake.

The second set of chapters set in the post-war period show the rapidly evolving nature of American psychiatry and the effect of the Mental Health Act on the evolution of psychiatric thinking and the impact of a growing "race neutrality." In an attempt to overcome the scientific racism of previous conceptions of the African American psyche, several practitioners, including an emerging cadre of African American psychiatrists, attempted to argue that the African American was no different in their susceptibility to mental illness, and therefore should be no different in their receipt of treatment. The implications of this shift are profound, as Doyle contends. On the one hand, race neutrality was designed to humanize the African American and to argue for equality in treatment. This argument underpinned the Civil Rights movement itself and was the basis for Kenneth and Mamie Clark's ground-breaking work on the importance of integrated education. At the same time, however, race neutral language (following a biomedical model) tended to "biologize" mental illness and therefore to render invisible the social structures which continued to affect the life chances of African Americans. What the psychiatrists in Doyle's book failed to understand (and what American psychiatry still struggles to address) is the connection between structures of oppression and the traumatizing effects of everyday racism on the human psyche. Doyle attempts to address this issue in his conclusion, but notes there is a long way to go.

The painstaking historical detail in this book, and the complicated arguments it makes, reflect the complexity of American psychiatry's relationship with race. In Doyle's book, we see the way in which the patient, in relation to race, is the entirety of African American communities, where those communities are posed as a problem. Yet the "treatment," ironically, is aimed at the individual. What is missing from the programs that Doyle documents is a sense of the desire for and outcomes of psychiatric help on the part of African Americans themselves. And this voice is missing from the book too, although not necessarily through any fault of the author, who clearly documents the paternalism inherent to white psychiatry and the difficulty of black practitioners themselves to be taken seriously. Indeed, the patients' voice is almost always missing in psychiatric histories, because the records themselves are often silent in this regard. As historians of psychiatry, we must always be cognizant of the way in which our study of programs, people, and ideas cannot really tell us anything about the lived experience of people with mental illness, and that we must work harder to make room for those voices. At the same time, Doyle's work is the third history of psychological or psychiatric services in Harlem. One could be forgiven for thinking that African Americans elsewhere did not experience mental illness, but of course this is not the case. Rather, this focus reflects the "social" nature of American psychiatry in the post-war period and its use in relation to highly visible social problems. The story of racist psychiatry outside the northern city remains largely to be told.

Notes

1. Jay Garcia, *Psychology Comes to Harlem: Rethinking the Race Question in Twentieth-Century America* (Baltimore, MD: Johns Hopkins University Press, 2012); Gabriel N. Mendes, *Under the Strain of Color: Harlem's Lafargue Clinic and the Promise of an Antiracist Psychiatry* (Ithaca, NY: Cornell University Press, 2015); Jonathan Metzl, *The Protest Psychosis: How Schizophrenia Became a Black Disease* (Boston, MA: Beacon Press, 2010); Mical Raz, *What's Wrong with the Poor? Psychiatry, Race and the War on Poverty* (Chapel Hill: University of North Carolina Press, 2013).

2. Sander Gilman, "On the Nexus of Blackness and Madness," in *Difference and Pathology: Sterotypes of Sexuality, Race and Madness* (Ithaca, NY: Cornell University Press, 1985), 131–149; John Hoberman, *Black and Blue: The Origins and Consequences of Medical Racism* (Berkeley: University of California Press, 2012); Khalil Gibran Muhammad, *The Condemnation of Blackness: Race, Crime and the Making of Modern Urban America* (Cambridge, MA: Harvard University Press, 2010); Daryl Michael Scott, *Contempt and Pity: Social Policy and the Image of the Damaged Black Psyche 1880–1996* (Chapel Hill: University of North Carolina Press, 1997).

KYLIE M. SMITH, PhD
Assistant Professor
Andrew W. Mellon Faculty Fellow for Nursing and the Humanities
Nell Hodgson Woodruff School of Nursing
Emory University

Birth Control in the Decolonizing Caribbean: Reproductive Politics and Practice on Four Islands, 1930–1970

By Nicole C. Bourbonnais
(Cambridge, UK: Cambridge University Press, 2016)
(253 pages; $99.00 hardcover)

Why study the history of birth control in four Caribbean islands? As historian Nicole Bourbonnais explains, the negotiations to promote birth control on the islands offer a perspective on how the struggle for reproductive rights might play out worldwide. The author asks that we abandon depictions of omnipotent imperialists and those of empowered local agents forging their own paths. Bourbonnais argues that birth control programs' past trajectories and future reproductive rights advocacy must acknowledge the larger world context, national political climates, community attitudes, and individual constraints.

The book's chapters follow the highly contested process of establishing birth control clinics in Bermuda, Barbados, Jamaica, and Trinidad. Running along a parallel track are external factors such as changes in the British Colonial Office's policies toward the Caribbean, the international movement for birth control, World War II, to name a few.

Bourbonnais places her study as part of both political and social history with transnational networks as a third slot in her historiographic framework, using class, gender, and race as analytical tools. Bourbonnais gathers a wealth of documents to support her multivariate perspective, tapping into archives on all four islands, Great Britain, and the international organizations that played key roles in discussing and implementing birth control at that time.

Chapter 1 focuses on "the intersection of transnational currents with local realities" (p. 31). The first debates on overpopulation in the islands appear in the context of the worldwide depression and protests against Great Britain's neglect of its colonies. Recommendations ranged from instructive pamphlets on contraception to compulsory sterilization for parents of "illegitimate" children; the outraged reactions reached the entire globe, thanks to expatriate Caribbean communities and to members of the transnational Pan-African movement. Many asserted that imperial authorities used overpopulation as a diversion to avoid economic and political reforms.

Nursing History Review 27 (2019): 128–130. A Publication of the American Association for the History of Nursing. Copyright © 2019 Springer Publishing Company.
http://dx.doi.org/10.1891/1062-8061.27.128

Chapter 2 explores why the Colonial Office, immersed in Malthusian discourses, failed to take significant measures against population growth it saw as "central cause of the poverty" on the islands. The author introduces the activists in the international birth control movement as a new set of non-state actors; but these visitors, just like the Colonial Office, did little to promote the birth control agenda given the scarcity of funding and local opposition wielding religious and race-suicide arguments.

In spite of resistance, birth control clinics opened between the late 1930s (first in Bermuda, 1939) and the mid-1950s. However, these were primarily privately funded, with little support from government. Chapter 3 examines the local reception to these clinics, paying close attention to individual testimonies of those who requested, received, or rejected these services. Bourbonnais excels at telling us why these women sought help, why they walked away, why they sometimes became ardent birth control advocates. She also highlights the indispensable role that nurses played in the success of some clinics, thanks to their identification with the patients and their commitment to helping the communities.

In the 1960s, global discourse shifted from birth control to family planning, hand-in-hand with Cold War theories of development, and spurring the creation of international aid organizations. Chapter 4 follows two lines of inquiry by looking at the interplay of international aid (through the United Nations, World Health Organization, United States Agency for International Development, and others) and local politicians seeking expansion of family planning programs.

Decolonization and independence in the British Caribbean allowed leaders sensitive to the need for both reduced population growth and systemic economic reforms to reach positions of power. These men and women were also aware of how controversies over birth control could affect their careers, and were ready to negotiate with opponents both radical and conservative. Independent governments were eligible to receive massive amounts of international funding for family planning endeavors, over which (the author claims) local groups were able to exercise control beyond the international donors' requirements.

Bourbonnais gives us a solidly documented narrative of how reproductive policies and programs are effectively implemented at the grassroots level, away from meeting rooms and congressional floors, as well as a detailed picture of the myriad moving parts involved in going from an abstract debate to a project for women, families, and communities. Her well-placed comparisons between other countries' programs make this book an excellent text for courses in international public health, nursing history, or histories of empire. The never smooth flow from population growth to birth control to family planning in the decades between 1930 and 1970 jumps out from the pages of the book and into our daily news, reminding us of the tasks ahead for the concept of reproductive rights to become a reality.

NEICI M. ZELLER, PhD
Associate Professor
History Department
William Paterson University
Wayne, NJ

Gender, Medicine, and Society in Colonial India: Women's Healthcare in Nineteenth- and Early Twentieth-Century Bengal

Sujata Mukherjee
(New Delhi, India: Oxford University Press, 2017)
(223 pages; $59.95 hardcover)

The complexity and vastness of Indian society requires examination from multiple viewpoints and even then the surface can barely be scratched. Florence Nightingale's extensive activity devoted to public health in Colonial India is not mentioned in Sujata Mukherjee's thoroughly researched book describing women and health care in colonial Bengal. Women's lot, possibly living in purdah, at times considered "unclean," and always subservient to men, made their access to medical care difficult at best. This is a story that will increase global understanding among historians of health care. Mukherjee's point was to examine gender and medicine within colonial India from the late 18th century until India's independence from Britain in 1947.

Mukherjee uses extensive primary and secondary sources to tease out the hidden life of women in India during these years. Prostitutes confined to the "Lock Hospitals" of the British Army were documented because of their integral role in the soldiers' health. Wealthier women who tried to secure an education or even a medical degree, left some tangible records of their presence. But the fate of the masses of Indian women, illiterate and poor, Mukherjee reconstructs from mortality tables and the descriptions of visiting female missionaries.

Issues of race, gender, and class are examined within this social history of medicine. The alleged superiority of Western medicine, Mukherjee argues, gave the British rulers an element of justification for their occupation. Her book opens with the hospitals, established around 1805, where Indian women suffering from venereal diseases were confined and treated. Following the Contagious Diseases Act of 1868 women working as prostitutes registered as such and entered these Lock Hospitals for regular examinations. Mukherjee wryly notes that the prostitutes were the "perpetrators" of venereal disease and the soldiers were the "victims." Later, around 1840, institutional care for those women desperate enough to be treated by male physicians included lying-in hospitals. Few women availed themselves of

Nursing History Review 27 (2019): 131–133. A Publication of the American Association for the History of Nursing. Copyright © 2019 Springer Publishing Company.
http://dx.doi.org/10.1891/1062-8061.27.131

these facilities. Over the course of the 19th-century, general hospitals and dispensaries opened but few women were admitted as patients. Trained female nurses are mentioned within the Calcutta hospitals of the mid-19th century. The obstacles confronting women who aspired to the practice of medicine were immense in a country where women's basic education was almost non-existent until the latter half of the 19th century. However, Mukherjee describes the intense need for female physicians in a country where women could not or would not see a male doctor. Some Hindu women used a female intermediary to interact with a doctor they never saw. In 1875, four women of European or Anglo-Indian origin entered the Madras Medical College as students, well before most European countries allowed women to train as doctors.

Written materials dealing with pre- and post-natal care and general health were another way to instruct the masses of Indian women in Western medical care. These educational tracts were written in the vernacular and encouraged women to turn away from the traditional lower-caste birth attendants, the dhais. Starting in the 1870s, European-style training for midwives was started at some teaching hospitals for women able to speak English—thus not the traditional dhais. Similarities between the denigration and eventual ouster of "Granny Midwives" in the United States and their Indian dhai counterparts are apparent. In her later chapters, Mukherjee addresses early 20th-century initiatives designed to promote the nation's health and, in many cases, to support India's nationalistic struggle. These included raising the marriageable age for girls, pre- and post-natal care, birth control, and eugenics. The Child Marriage Restraint Act of 1929 raised the age of permissible sexual intercourse within marriage from 12 to 14. Large employers in Bengal, such as tea growers, started maternity and child welfare benefits for their employees; others employed company midwives for their workers. Birth control and eugenics movements were partially fueled by concern over population increases and a desire to "improve the race, and eliminate the 'unfit'" (p. 135). Mukherjee then describes the impact on women of the 1943–1944 Bengal famine, exacerbated by their poverty, their diet, and diseases such as tuberculosis. Her description of the state of the victims, well supported by data, is sobering. Mukherjee concludes her work with the closing years of the British occupation of India and assessments of women's health as the country re-entered a state of independence.

From the perspective of a US nurse historian, Mukherjee has provided a valuable account of an under-studied group and their access to health care. The millions of women seen through her painstaking research, women hidden because of purdah or caste, were illuminating. Mukherjee's book would be useful for a graduate student or researcher interested in the field of global women's health in the 19th century.

BRIGID LUSK, PHD
Adjunct Clinical Professor
College of Nursing
University of Illinois at Chicago

Bellevue: Three Centuries of Medicine and Mayhem at America's Most Storied Hospital

By David Oshinsky
(New York: Doubleday, 2016)
(387 pages; $20.40 cloth, $11.59 paper, $12.99 e-book).

David Oshinsky's *Bellevue: Three Centuries of Medicine and Mayhem at America's Most Storied Hospital* provides an evocative insight into one of New York's most celebrated institutions. Oshinsky captures New York City's most noted municipal hospital's very essence that has followed it throughout its history, which is serving the poor, the immigrants, and the gravely injured. In telling the story of Bellevue, he tells the story of the history of medicine noting several firsts at Bellevue, including a municipal ambulance corps, advances in surgery, use of anesthesia, forensics, and medical education.

Oshinsky organizes the book around some of the ways in which Bellevue addressed their commitment to caring for the vulnerable populations of New York City. Early chapters reflect the vision of city leaders to provide an almshouse and prison for its citizens in the then northern outskirts of New York City along the East River. Tracing its history back to the 1600s—this revered outpost for the medically indigent evolved overtime as it moved uptown to its present site along the East River. This hospital, as Oshinksy describes it "…has born witness to every imaginable disease and public health scare, every economic swing and population surge, every medical breakthrough and controversy going back more than two centuries" (p. 5). Each chapter presents one of these stories, placing its history squarely within the context of the day. Care of the immigrants, the Irish, Germans, and Italians in the late 19th and early 20th century, gave way to more recent immigration from Haitians, Hispanics, Africans, South Asians, and Chinese. Race, class, and gender, while not specifically signaled out, were reflected throughout the history of this hospital, the people it cared for, and those that provided care. For example, in a city where the other early medical schools—New York Hospital and Columbia, summarily rejected Jews and African Americans, Bellevue offered opportunity.

Medical care, more primitive in the early days of Bellevue, lacked the benefit of the germ theory, or even the use of anesthesia. Care during epidemics that plagued the city tell a story of commitment by the physicians and the city itself where it turned no one away—unlike other hospitals that

Nursing History Review 27 (2019): 134–137. A Publication of the American Association for the History of Nursing. Copyright © 2019 Springer Publishing Company.
http://dx.doi.org/10.1891/1062-8061.27.134

opened in New York. Oshinksy contrasts the history of these other voluntary- and religious-based hospitals, describing that Bellevue did not and could not turn any person in need away. Care during the many epidemics that plagued the city—small pox in the 1700s, yellow fever ("Yellow Jack") in the 1800s, influenza pandemic in 1918, HIV in the later part of the 20th century, and the more recent outbreak of Ebola—showed the enduring commitment to all in need. Oshinsky provides an account of Bellevue's care of mental illness, a history that remains steadfast in popular memory. While psychiatric care was mostly observational, it nevertheless became and perhaps continues to be closely associated with Bellevue's name and reputation.

The book reflects Bellevue's response to emergencies, whether to victims of crime, terrorism, or natural disasters. Considered another one of its "firsts" was a chapter devoted to the Bellevue Ambulance, where following the Civil War, it came to be recognized that a "rapid response" like the one initiated on the battlefield to remove wounded soldiers was needed to care for civilians where they fell in the streets. Oshinsky writes that Dalton, the physician who championed ambulance corps in New York gave an example comparing the neglect of soldiers to when "an exhausted workingman who had fallen from a streetcar one night near the Battery, the southern tip of New York" (p. 113). When no one was able to find a horse and wagon to carry him safely uptown to Bellevue for several hours, the man died enroute.

Other firsts integrated in various chapters included the evolution of medical education along with the introduction of advances in science that enhanced the work of physicians. Simple handwashing and the eventual use of rubber gloves during surgeries and the care of mothers' in labor significantly reduced the mortality from the ever present risk of infection.

To his credit, Oshinsky includes a chapter on nursing, titled, Nightingales. This chapter briefly outlines the beginning of the nurse training school at Bellevue. Oshinsky gives a history of Nightingale's contribution in the Crimean and her influence on nursing education in England. Although Nightingale was not a proponent of the germ theory (a bit before her time), she supported the notion of a clean air, good food, pure water as ways in which to reduce mortality and morbidity. Oshinsky speaks of her use of "mortality diagrams" to help explain the better outcomes she observed following improvement of the hospital environment. Her work influenced the new school to open at Bellevue in 1873 and considered among one of Bellevue's long list of "firsts." This same chapter provides context for changes in maternity care—where the simple act of washing hands could reduce the loss of life—both mother and baby—from puerperal fever. The new nursing school brought a "sense of order that spread within the crumbling shells of the buildings, reminiscent of Nightingale in Crimea" (p. 139). Oshinsky briefly mentions the beginning of a school for men in nursing at Bellevue and a scandal related to the male nurses. This could be this reviewer's bias, however, as I wish there had been a more comprehensive history of this notable Bellevue "first." It seemed to be a stand-alone chapter. Rather than integrating nursing education, as it did medical education throughout the book, nurses, and nursing education seems to be paternalistically taken for granted—something that was expected of women and just part of the daily fabric of the hospital. While the other chapters placed Bellevue within the context of New York's political, social, and economic history, there was no mention of Bellevue's nurses working in public health (something the book addressed) or community ventures on the lower east side of New York. For example, no mention of Lillian Wald's efforts with caring for the same immigrant population that Bellevue cared for. There also was nothing about Bellevue's consistent leadership in nursing education like the early decision to phase out its diploma based program and enter the world of baccalaureate and higher degree education. The book, while omitting this one relevant story to the history of Bellevue and health care, it is a great read that had a great deal of material to cover, and only one volume to fill.

Oshinsky tells the story using several archives, oral histories, and historiographies to support his work. What I found difficult to follow is where he cites his references, perhaps because of the style that the publisher uses. The references used do reflect a wide array of sources. But a weakness I noted in the chapter on nursing was that there was no reference to the Bellevue Hospital School of Nursing archives at the NY Foundation of Nurses in Guilderland, New York. Not a fatal flaw, but perhaps, that is why the story of Bellevue's leadership played in the nursing education and practice was underplayed and seemingly omitted. However, what it does show is how the use of different source materials, interpreted from different perspectives, offer different historical stories.

Oshinsky narrates a great story about Bellevue and the many changes it underwent reflecting improvements in science, advances in education, and expanding urban environments. Throughout the years, Oshinsky showed Bellevue's continued commitment to the health and well-being of the people of New York City. Those interested in the history of medicine, the history of New York City, and health care in general would enjoy this interesting and informative book.

SANDRA B. LEWENSON, EdD, RN, FAAN
Professor
College of Health Professions
Lienhard School of Nursing
Pace University
133 Mt. Hope Blvd.
Hastings-on-Hudson, NY 10706

Deaconesses in Nursing Care: International Transfer of a Female Model of Life and Work in the 19th and 20th Century

Edited by Susanne Kreutzer and Karen Nolte
(Stuttgart, Germany: Franz Steiner Verlag, 2016) (230 pages; $69.00 paper)

In what editors Susanne Kreutzer and Karen Nolte describe as a *transnational history*, the work of Lutheran deaconess nurses in the 19th and 20th centuries is illuminated. This collection of multifaceted essays resulted from an international colloquium of history scholars at Kaiserswerth in 2013. Collectively, the authors share a global perspective contributing to what is known about the Lutheran deaconess history spanning two centuries. Previous studies speak to the transfer of deaconess communities to other parts of the world with an emphasis on formal education and nursing care. No other text addresses to what extent the German model was adapted considering the variable social and political factors influencing the Lutheran deaconess work in the international context of care provision in Palestine, Scandinavia, England, and the United States.

The *transnational* approach to history provides a useful framework for the study of the Lutheran deaconess movement and the subsequent transfer of ideas from Germany to other parts of the world. Much of this transfer was due to benevolent religious organizations that came to the aid of the sick and poor because of nonexistent or limited social programs before 1900. Contributing author Annett Büttner captured this idea suggesting the "international spread of the deaconess organization can be likened to not-for-profit franchising" (p. 37). It was impassioned clergy and denominational leadership who borrowed from the German Lutheran deaconess model to transplant formal education and nursing to care for parishioners and others in their communities.

The first section of the book speaks to the foundation of the Lutheran deaconess movement. Karen Nolte provides a concise overview of the German deaconess motherhouse and the formal education of young women to include religious and practical nurse training begun in 1836 by Lutheran pastor Theodor Fliedner. Matthias Honold draws from a case study describing the successful transfer of German deaconess work to Neuendettelsau established in 1854 by Wilhelm Löhe. It was identified that the motherhouse model of accommodation versus a stand-alone training school was a necessary compo-

Nursing History Review 27 (2019): 138–140. A Publication of the American Association for the History of Nursing. Copyright © 2019 Springer Publishing Company.
http://dx.doi.org/10.1891/1062-8061.27.138

nent for success. Löhe also developed principles of nursing incorporating care of both body and soul. Annett Büttner examines denomination based males and females providing nursing care on the battlefields of the Danish German War of 1864. With a dearth of military medical service, Lutherans and Catholics put aside theological differences to meet the needs of the wounded. This model provided a template for the development of future secular models of volunteer nurses.

In the second section of the book, two essays illustrate Lutheran *Outer Mission* in Jerusalem. Authors Uwe Kaminsky and Ruth Wexler speak to Fliedner's original plan of recruiting more women to the deaconess work; however, this plan was not to be realized. While the German deaconesses achieved their aim in the providing care to the community and in a home for lepers, the work was not self-sustaining over time.

The third section speaks to the successful transfer of the German model to the Scandinavian countries of Denmark, Sweden, and Finland. Susanne Dietz investigates the Kaiserswerth General Conference organized by Fliedner in 1861 to bring together a worldwide organization of deaconess motherhouses. Conference records provide a careful accounting of numbers of motherhouses, deaconesses, and fields of activity reported over time. Considerable growth occurred from 1860 to 1913 when the onset of World War I greatly changed perceptions and social structures. Dietz argues that the success of the deaconess movement depended upon religious conditions and the strength (or lack thereof) of the motherhouse. Pirjo Markkola describes how the German model flourished in Finland particularly in the community setting where parish deaconesses cared for both body and soul. As municipal poor relief systems were created in the changing social structure in the 20th century, the role of the church in community outreach needed to be reconsidered. The work of the deaconess became the precursor to paid public health and visiting nurses.

The final chapters illuminate the transfer to the United Kingdom and the United States as well as limitations of the deaconess work. Carmen Mangion uses two case studies as evidence of the significance of Kaiserswerth "as a hub to a transnational deaconess movement" in England. The Kaiserswerth model met with early success in faith based hospitals and in the community with parish deaconesses; however, by the 1900s, with the growing needs of a complex medical marketplace, religious nurses were replaced by hospital-trained nurses. The push for professionalization of nursing took center stage. Doris Riemann captures a history of the transfer of the deaconess model to the United States in Baltimore 1895 and extending to the 1960s. While there was early success, the changing social landscape, the push for professionalism, efficiency, and standardization, along with expanding roles for women resulted in an obsolete model. Women sought independent accommodation, regular wages, and working hours. In the final essay of the text, Kreutzer provides a comprehensive conclusion for the transnational history of nursing, medicine, religion, gender, and social influences.

Kreutzer and Nolte make a significant contribution to the Lutheran deaconess history offering both historical and more contemporary perspectives of the evolution and formalization of nurse education as well as the transfer of ideas from the German Lutheran deaconesses to other countries. The research is well supported by the extensive primary and secondary sources explored by the contributing authors. Several audiences will find this text of interest. Historians focused on 19th- and 20th-century nursing and education will come away with a better understanding of the German Lutheran diaspora of ideas. Community clergy and others will find this history of interest from a denominational perspective. Those exploring in a transnational historical approach will find this framework useful for application. The contemporary parish nurse, now called faith community nurse, will come away with a better understanding of the historical foundation of wholistic care of body and spirit.

LISA M. ZERULL, PhD, RN-BC
Adjunct Nursing Faculty
Faith Community Nurse
Grace Evangelical Lutheran Church
339 Green Spring Drive
Winchester, VA 22603

Toxic Histories: Poison and Pollution in Modern India

By David Arnold
(Cambridge: Cambridge University Press, 2016)
(241 pages; $42.78 cloth, $17.50 paper, $40.00 e-book)

David Arnold's *Toxic Histories* narrates the "long history of India's toxic entanglements" (p. 208). It is neither a history of poisons nor toxicology. Rather it addresses "in equal measure the social cognition and scientific understanding of poisons and poisoning in nineteenth and twentieth century India" (p. 3). It speaks in turns to the history of medicine, history of science—especially the histories of toxicology and forensics, but also the histories of chemistry, botany, and so forth, the history of environmental pollution, and of course the history of colonial power.

Arnold makes three inter-related arguments in the book. First, he posits that India has had a particularly complex and long set of historical associations with both ideas and materials of toxicity. With the possible exception of China, the range of India's historical, cultural, and material associations with poisons, he contends, is unrivalled (p. 209). Second, he argues that around the cusp of the 19th and 20th centuries, India underwent a "toxic transition." This transition entailed "a shift from state-centered preoccupations with person-specific, poison related crime to the growing concerns of a middle-class Indian public ... with the poisoning ... from adulterated foods and unregulated drugs..." (p. 15). Third, the generalized public concern with toxicity eventually leads to a recalibration of the urban Indian milieu, namely its airs, waters and foods, as potentially "toxic."

These key arguments are advanced alongside several minor arguments and a wealth of riveting tales in the course of seven chapters, an introduction and a conclusion. The first chapter establishes the pre-colonial backdrop in which the rest of the narrative unfolds. Arnold discusses the mythological, the medical, and the sociological lives of poisons in pre-colonial India in this opening chapter. In Chapter 2, he proceeds to outline the early 19th-century botanical and chemical attempts by the imperialists to discover, tame, and exploit Indian poisons. Rather than mineral poisons, which dominated European discourses on the subject, in India Arnold finds that, with the exception of arsenic, it was mainly the three vegetable poisons, that is, aconite, datura, and opium, which engaged imperial attention. Snake venom of course was another imperial preoccupation and it too is briefly discussed.

Nursing History Review 27 (2019): 141–143. A Publication of the American Association for the History of Nursing. Copyright © 2019 Springer Publishing Company.
http://dx.doi.org/10.1891/1062-8061.27.141

In Chapter 3, these imperial concerns take on a more sinister tone as Arnold inaugurates a discussion of the imperial anxieties over being poisoned. Much of the chapter discusses the case of the Robert Phayre, the British Resident to the court of Baroda, and his allegations that the reigning Gaekwad monarch, Malharrao, tried to poison him in November 1874 using crushed diamonds. The next chapter moves into a history of forensic science in India. It recounts the toxicological knowledge in early medical jurisprudence and the emergence of the office of the Chemical Examiners. Chapter 5 is a page-turner, devoted to the intimate crimes where poison was used or thought to have been used. The bulk of the chapter is devoted to the Agra Double Murder Case of 1911 when a European woman and a Eurasian doctor, involved in an adulterous affair, murdered both their respective spouses. Arnold shows not only how poison panics such as the Agra Case connected the intimate domestic spaces to public discourses, but also how the ambiguities of racial politics over-determined these panics. The following chapter explores how poisons were gradually "embraced," that is, as medicines, as pesticides, and so forth. This chapter also charts the relocation of toxic associations away from the Indian society at large and onto the lower-caste subaltern orders. Finally, Chapter 7 charts how Indian and British scientists converge in reclassifying many elements of the urban Indian environment as "toxic." Arnold calls this the expansion of the penumbra of poisons, that is, a discrete idea of poisons begins to inflate and blur into a much wider, diffuse notion. This is where poison increasingly shades into pollution. In the brief conclusion, Arnold goes further and notices much continuity between the late colonial and postcolonial periods. He also provocatively asks whether some of the limited controls mechanisms, put in place during the early 20th century for regulating urban toxicity, were not over-hastily dismantled in the wake of the postcolonial enthusiasm for rapid industrial growth, leading to an often toxic present (p. 208).

The book is lucidly written and refreshingly free of any jargon. Stories abound and the narrative seldom lags. The book's key arguments are provocative and the associations Arnold makes are far from obvious. Traditional historians will undoubtedly feel Arnold moves too quickly from one topic to another, but it is precisely the lateral connections which make the book so much more than a mere cultural history of toxicity. Crucial to the book's aspirations is the insight that there is a fundamental ambiguity enshrined at the heart of the classical idea of the *pharmakon*, whereby a substance can both be a life-saving medicine and a life-taking toxicant depending on the context. Poisons operate by unsettling and disturbing fixed categories. *Toxic Histories*, too, aims to unsettle.

At only slightly over 200 pages, *Toxic Histories* is not a comprehensive history of any single topic. It is rather a fascinating argument about a range of topics threaded together by a series of well-told, gripping tales. It is neither definitive nor exhaustive, but it is most certainly inspiring and inciting.

PROJIT BIHARI MUKHARJI, PhD
Associate Professor
History & Sociology of Science
University of Pennsylvania

Children and Drug Safety: Balancing Risk and Protection in Twentieth-Century America

By Cynthia A. Connolly
(New Brunswick, NJ: Rutgers University Press, 2018)
(260 pages; $37.95 paper, $99.95 cloth, $37.95 e-book)

Historians of medicine and pharmacy have shown increasing interest recently in the history of pharmaceuticals, with books on the subject published within the last 10 years by Scott Podolsky, Jeremey Greene, Dominique Tobbell, David Herzberg, Andrea Tone, and other scholars. There has been one aspect of the topic, however, that has received almost no attention from historians, namely, the use of medicines in children. Now Cynthia Connolly's *Children and Drug Safety: Balancing Risk and Protection in Twentieth-Century America* admirably fills that gap in the literature.

Connolly skillfully weaves together the strands of pharmaceutical, medical, and nursing history, as well as changing views of child development and regulatory control of drugs, to tell the fascinating story of drug therapeutics and policy for children in the United States in the 20th century. She begins with concerns over the widespread use of opiate-laced soothing syrups for babies in the late 19th and early 20th centuries and carries the history up through the 1970s, with a brief epilogue chapter on "Pediatric Drug Development and Policy after 1979." Along the way, she discusses such important developments as the use of antibiotics in children, the concept of the therapeutic orphan, the problem of baby aspirin poisoning, marketing of drugs for children, and pediatric psychopharmacology. Throughout the book, Connolly analyzes the continuing tensions and interactions between physicians (especially pediatricians), the Food and Drug Administration, the pharmaceutical industry, and parents.

Connolly corrects the mistaken view expressed by some authors that children and pregnant women were routinely excluded from drug studies before the 1970s. As she explains:

> In researching this book, I learned that at some historical moments it had been considered in children's best interest for them to participate in drug trials, sometimes with their parents' knowledge, sometime without it. At different historical junctures, children were barred from such research in an effort to protect them. In other words, the ethics regarding how best to evaluate drugs in the pediatric population has been dynamic and contingent. (p. 5)

Nursing History Review 27 (2019): 144–146. A Publication of the American Association for the History of Nursing. Copyright © 2019 Springer Publishing Company.
http://dx.doi.org/10.1891/1062-8061.27.144

The difficulties of determining whether or not particular drugs act the same way in children as they do in adults, and of establishing appropriate dosages for children at various age levels, is a continuing theme throughout the book. For example, in the 1930s, it was discovered that amphetamines calmed children with behavior disorders, rather than acting as a stimulant as they did in adults. Physicians have long recognized that calculating a suitable dose of a drug for a child based on weight, as compared to an adult, could result in an overdose, with possible serious consequences, or an ineffective dose. They struggled, however, with coming up with suitable alternatives. Clearly more clinical trials with children were called for, but the pharmaceutical industry resisted paying for these as in their view the costs of getting new drugs approved had already skyrocketed under increased regulation. There were also complicated ethical concerns involved in testing drugs on children. Consequently, many drugs were marketed with instructions that they had not been approved for use in children, leaving physicians on their own to decide whether or not to administer a drug to a child and what the appropriate dose should be. Even today these issues have not been fully addressed, as Connolly points out.

Another prominent theme is the marketing of drugs for children. The pharmaceutical industry did not view children as a significant market before the 1930s, as many physicians believed that drugs offered more risk than benefit in children. With the introduction of the sulfonamides, followed by the antibiotics, the use of drug therapy in children dramatically increased. Drug firms became interested in developing formulations of these drugs that would appeal to children, for example, flavored syrups. It was an attempt to produce a version of sulfanilamide palatable to children that led to the Elixir of Sulfanilamide disaster in 1937. The development of baby aspirin is an especially illuminating and interesting example of marketing of drugs aimed at children, and Connolly devotes a chapter to this subject. In 1947, St. Joseph Aspirin for Children, an orange-flavored chewable tablet, was introduced onto the market the first of a number of similar products. Although this product made it easier for parents to get their children to take aspirin, it also caused a dramatic increase in aspirin poisoning among children. In a sense, the manufacturer was too successful in developing a palatable product, as children loved the taste of what came to be referred to as candy aspirin. Industry, concerned about losing sales, resisted attempts to reduce poisoning by safety-caps, warning labels, or discontinuing the use of flavoring, placing the blame on careless parents who did not adequately supervise their children.

Connolly skillfully discusses all of these issues and more, providing new perspectives and insights. *Children and Drug Safety* is too complex and rich a work for me to cover all of its themes and conclusions in a review. It is well written and meticulously researched, drawing on a host of archival and published sources. Historians of various fields, health professionals and policy makers would all benefit from reading this book.

JOHN PARASCANDOLA, PhD
Public Health Service Historian (Retired)
Bethesda, MD

The End of Physiotherapy

David A. Nicholls
(London and New York: Routledge, 2017)
(286 pages; $140.00 hardcover)

David Nicholls' *The End of Physiotherapy* is a unique monograph in many respects. An Australian physical therapist of 30 years who also holds a PhD in philosophy, Nicholls provides a historical and theoretical survey of his own oft-overlooked allied health profession. The author makes clear from the outset that the audience for his book is "practitioners, students, teachers, researchers and those who work to shape the profession's future" (p. 4). As the title makes clear, Nicholls feels a sense of urgency about the potential demise of his profession worldwide. An advocate of the importance of his trade, Nicholls worries that the profession is still unthinkingly wedded to its early 20th-century formative years, and thus unprepared to face the post-welfare-state that is emerging in the 21st century.

The book is divided into three parts. The first section covers the 100 years history of physiotherapy, charting the field's World War I beginnings in the United States, Britain, and the Commonwealth down to the present day. Crucial to Nicholls' periodization is the 1973 oil crisis, when neoliberal forces began to dismantle the welfare state, and its robust health care system. Part II offers a critical analysis of key biomedical assumptions of physiotherapy—that is, notions of the body, functional movement, and rehabilitation—that undergird the profession's practice and education. The last section gestures toward changes in physiotherapy education, regulation, practice, and policy that Nicholls thinks would ensure the continuation of the field.

Non-specialists have the most to gain from the historical and critical analysis that Nicholls provides. Only a handful of scholars (myself included) have attended to the history of physical therapy, and Nicholls makes an extremely persuasive case that far more work needs to be done. A PhD-PT myself, I am particularly sympathetic to his frustration with the lack of historical and philosophical self-consciousness among practitioners. Physiotherapy, he argues, has been "a profession that mirrors dominant white, European culture in that it assumes that culture is something others have and that there is 'objective' truth to the biomedical—or more accurately biomechanical—basis to the profession's practice that does not need to be questioned. It just *is*" (p. 5, emphasis in original).

Nursing History Review 27 (2019): 147–149. A Publication of the American Association for the History of Nursing. Copyright © 2019 Springer Publishing Company.
http://dx.doi.org/10.1891/1062-8061.27.147

More specifically, physiotherapy's adherence to understanding the body-as-machine, Nicholls argues, has led to a kind of reductionism and mind–body dualism that excludes "other cultural, environmental, humanistic, spiritual or social understandings of the body" (p. 17). The author demonstrates that while adopting such an understanding of the body was necessary a century ago to legitimize the field in the eyes of orthodox medicine and the public, it is not well suited for a neoliberal 21st century, where the welfare state is crumbling under austerity measures and health is increasingly understood as an individual pursuit of patients as "consumers" who view their own bodies in myriad ways. If physiotherapy is to remain current, he continues, it needs to teach its practitioners to look at the whole patient and to see the body as a multiplicity, "a tool," a "spiritual envelop," an "existence," an "art form," a "personal identity" (p. 132).

As a work of history, *The End of Physiotherapy*, relies more on secondary sources than new archival finds, and the narrative encompasses too many regions of the globe to adequately satisfy scholarly standards expected of a professional historian. Nevertheless, Nicholls' argument about the ahistoricism of the profession is convincing, and he is at his best when engaging in Foucauldian-inspired analysis of what history and critical analysis means to the profession. Most provocatively, Nicholls argues that any field that cannot offer a critical history of itself is bound to die.

One may wonder, of course, what a more humanistic physiotherapist has to offer. Here, Nicholls seems to be more concerned with the longevity of his own profession than he is with improving patient care or social justice (not that these are mutually exclusive). While Nicholls seems disillusioned with the neoliberal state, his advice for physiotherapists is to adapt to the new marketplace rather than fight against the health inequality it creates. With the dismantling of the welfare state, Nicholls contends that practitioners need to embrace a holistic view of the body, otherwise "they will lose patients. Consumers will abandon physiotherapy in favor of practitioners who celebrate [the consumer's] individuality and turn it into a virtue" (p. 107). In making such statements, Nicholls seems to shrink from the very point he wishes to make: namely, that physiotherapists are—and have been—too apolitical and unthinking. "Physiotherapists have been more interested in joint movements than social movements," he writes, "preferring to leave the planning and organization of health and welfare to others" (pp. 85–169). He complains that "rather than focusing on social determinants of health" (i.e., employment, diet, housing), physiotherapists have tended to focus on individual pathology (p. 90). And yet, *The End of Physiotherapy* encourages the very kind of political complacency that it wishes to critique, for the goal of displacing the view of the body-as-machine with a more "holistic" approach is, at base, a move driven by the market; it is an attempt to create a niche in the neoliberal world, where only a fraction of the population can afford physical therapy, thereby making it a luxury item, not a universal health care right.

While Nicholls' practical advice proves to be somewhat disappointing, this should not detract from his scholarly ambition to offer a critical analysis of the history and practice of physiotherapy, which is long overdue. *The End of Physiotherapy* is an ideal jumping off point for further humanistic research into the areas of manual therapy, rehabilitation, health care policy, and disability.

BETH LINKER, PHD
Associate Professor and Graduate Chair
History and Sociology of Science
University of Pennsylvania

Rise of the Modern Hospital: An Architectural History of Health and Healing, 1870–1940

By Jeanne Kisacky
(Pittsburgh, PA: University of Pittsburgh Press)
(448 pages; $65.00 hardcover, $51.99 e-book)

In *Notes on Hospitals*, Florence Nightingale noted that different hospitals treating the sick and injured had very different death and recovery rates.[1] For the remainder of her life, Nightingale applied her observations to influence the design of hundreds of hospitals in her hope of promoting health and preventing the spread of disease. In *Rise of the Modern Hospital*, Jeanne Kisacky sets out to explore how American hospital design "facilitated cure and suppressed illness" (p. 3) from the mid-19th to the mid-20th century in America. Over that period of time, the designers of American hospitals debated whether the hospital building was therapeutic in and of itself, or whether it was a tool to house the therapeutic process. This debate is relevant today, as designers of hospitals focus on building structures that are efficient, attractive, and increasingly patient-centered.

Examining historical buildings, as Kisacky does in *Rise of the Modern Hospital*, does reveal much about the intentions of the designers, and the activities of the occupants—including the patients, nurses, and physicians. While Kisacky is an architect and writes from that perspective, this work reveals much about the practice of American nursing and medicine in the time period studied. It also became apparent to this non-architect that the very language of hospital design and construction, so well documented in this work, is still used in hospitals and by healthcare providers today.

Kisacky starts with the early American hospitals designed on the European traditions, and based on the miasma theory of disease transmission. These early American hospital designers used Nightingale's hospital reform work to guide the design and construction of Pavilion-style hospitals, with wards that were designed to optimize natural light and fresh air. During this period, the healthful hospital site was as important as the structure. Hospitals were built away from city-centers, and the buildings had a large footprint on the site, as one to two story buildings were deemed best for circulation of fresh air and light. Even in this early period of American hospital design, architectural features such as the use of impervious hospital surfaces, rounded corners, and elaborate ventilation systems were used and well documented by Kisacky.

Nursing History Review 27 (2019): 150–152. A Publication of the American Association for the History of Nursing. Copyright © 2019 Springer Publishing Company.
http://dx.doi.org/10.1891/1062-8061.27.150

After the adoption of germ theory and the dawn of the age of antisepsis, the goal of the hospital designer was to build a "germ-proof" structure. While many hospitals from this era continued to use the Pavilion style as a foundation, the restriction on the number of hospital floors to improve ventilation was liberalized. Hospitals from this era, such as New York Hospital and Cook County Hospital in Chicago could be built closer to more densely populated areas of the city. As more floors were added to the building, the footprint became smaller and less acreage was needed for a new hospital site.

Hospital design over time was influenced by more than the understanding of infection transmission and asepsis. Race, gender, and class always influenced the ward design and patient ward assignment. Hospitals consistently added design features to attract paying patients, such as private rooms and specialty wards. At the end of the 19th century, new medical therapies, such as X-rays, surgery, and blood transfusions, demanded space within the new American hospital. In the late 19th and early 20th centuries, changes in medical education also influenced hospital design, and hospital-affiliated schools required space for classroom and clinical education. Dispensaries and clinics were added to hospitals to enhance the educational experience, and nurse-run specialty wards were added to attract high-quality (and high volume) physicians.

The first decades of the 20th century brought about the era of efficiency, and Kisacky describes the change in hospital configuration from "hygienic decentralization" to "functional centralization." Rather than having decentralized operating theaters for each specialty, centralized operating floors became the norm. Nursing shortages forced hospital directors to examine the "nurse travel distance" and the Nightingale ward was found to be grossly inefficient. To help reduce nurse fatigue, hospital designers incorporated labor-saving technologies and design features such as the dumbwaiter, the pneumatic tube system, and patient call lights. Many of these features to enhance nurse efficiency were most effective in hospitals that were organized vertically, rather than the expansive pavilion-style structures.

By the end of Kisacky's work, the transformation is complete. The American hospital, once viewed as "therapy," became the "attractive factory" for providing efficient medical care. Attention to environmental purification persisted; however, in contrast to the Nightingale era of fresh air and ventilation the early 20th-century hospitals focused on closed circulation. The modern hospital was "hermetically sealed" (p. 323) and the open window was viewed as archaic.

As noted, Kisacky is an architect and this book reflects that attention to architectural detail. However, this work does not ignore the professional, social, and economic factors that influenced the design of American hospitals from 1870 to 1940. It was easy to read this book as a nurse, picture the specific types of hospital design and imagine how the physical space would have impacted the care provided within the American hospital. The book is well researched, references many known publications examining the history of the hospital, and is heavily illustrated with pictures, plans, and drawings. *Rise of the Modern Hospital* is a rich and scholarly work, and a must read for anyone interested in the history of the American hospital.

Note

1. Florence Nightingale, *Notes on Hospitals—Primary Source Edition*, (London: Longman, Green, Longman, Roberts and Green, 1863).

BETH HUNDT, PHD, APRN
School of Nursing
University of Virginia
225 Jeanette Lancaster Way
Charlottesville, VA 22903

Nursing and Empire: Gendered Labor and Migration from India to the United States

By Sujani K. Reddy
(Chapel Hill, NC: University of North Carolina Press, 2015)
(290 pages; $32.95 paper, $26.99 e-book)

Unlike scientists, engineers, and physicians, nurses have been overlooked in professional labor migration from India to the United States. However, simply tacking nurses to the list is insufficient, Sujani Reddy notes. Rather, deeper analysis of Indian nurse migration to the United States reveals more complex problems surrounding immigration, gender, and class (p. 3). It also furthers our understanding of nursing's stratification and racialization. To encompass all of these issues, Reddy turns our attention to American imperialism. She demonstrates that this factor is essential to understanding Indian nurses immigrating and negotiating their place in American nursing and society.[1]

First, Reddy traces the beginnings of imperialism in India, then moves to analyzing Indian nurses' experiences in the United States. In Chapter 1, Reddy describes how Protestant missionaries evangelized to Indian women through teaching domestic skills. They established a gendered division of labor that foregrounded nursing's feminization. In Chapter 2, Reddy analyzes archives for international nursing leaders' intentional "civilizing mission," magnifying their underlying imperialistic attitudes (p. 57). These leaders trained India's first nurses, who were typically Christians and lower-caste laborers left to take on the "unclean" work of nursing (p. 47). In Chapters 3–5, Reddy outlines the Rockefeller Foundation's efforts to spread the biomedical approach to medicine through building new universities. These institutions produced India's own nursing leaders, whose education geared them more toward their benefactors' priorities and less so to India's health care needs. Not surprisingly, these nurses began to look toward the United States for career opportunities. In Chapter 6, Reddy synthesizes nursing history scholarship to establish the racialized stratification that Indian nurses entered in the United States. Many American nursing schools were still segregated, and working-class students were attracted to LPN and diploma programs that offered stipends and room and board. Nursing leaders worried that these programs watered down the standards of the profession. Indian nurses' place in this hierarchy became complicated

Nursing History Review 27 (2019): 153–155. A Publication of the American Association for the History of Nursing. Copyright © 2019 Springer Publishing Company.
http://dx.doi.org/10.1891/1062-8061.27.153

by their foreign status, which was later institutionalized through the Exchange Visitor Program, H-1 visas, and examinations for foreign-educated nurses.

Reddy's original interviews appear in the last parts of her book. In Chapter 7, she uses them to express nurses' difficulties working in the United States. Then in Chapter 8, the interviews capture their vexed status as both "women in the lead" and "women on the loose" (pp. 184–193). Indian nurses could gain work visas, making them the gateways for family reunification provisions in immigration law. And yet, these same women are seen as deviating from the male-dominated family structures that both Indian and American culture reinforces. This duality is perhaps one of the most important themes that Reddy addresses, as it unlocks her analysis of post-war immigration law, as well as of the Asian American model-minority myth. Furthermore, it complicates the more common female immigrant labor narrative of exploitation. Reddy's use of original interviews shines here, as her interviewees' words convey their ambivalent attitudes toward their status. Her deft interpretation of these interviews is also featured in Reddy's short but powerful epilogue.

The epilogue demonstrates the broader understanding that Reddy's analysis of imperialism allows as she gestures toward one last topic: Indian nurses' families—or rather, their different kinship structures, which, in some cases, deviate from the ideal American household of a mother and father with children. Instead, a few Indian women form households as single mothers or divorcees, or return to and provide for their natal families. After she arrives to the United States, a woman by the pseudonym Subhashini ends up living with a group of Indian immigrant physicians. They then help other Indian women who immigrate and re-establish their lives. Though they all have moved out, they continue to connect and reunite. Reddy treats these kinship structures not as aberrations or failures, but as "possibilities" of roles that Indian nurses can play for other women (p. 210). While Reddy had met numerous Indian nurses who were married with children, she notes these other possibilities that we, too, can see after considering immigration and American imperialism. This book will enlighten nursing scholars who are also interested in gender, Asian American studies, and professional labor migration.

Note

1. Reddy, 152. "[…] Indian im/migration was a product of a critical, cumulative history that had connected U.S.-based institutions and individuals to Indian nursing labor through the circuits of Anglo-American capitalist imperialism. While these ties were less readily apparent in India than for other nations topping the list, such as the Philippines and South Korea, they are nevertheless crucial for understanding how the workings of capitalist imperialism abroad affected the re-racialization of foreign nurse immigration to the United States during the Cold War."

ANDRE A. ROSARIO, BSN, RN
Penn Medicine Princeton Medical Center
One Plainsboro Road
Plainsboro, NJ 08536

A History of Global Health: Interventions into the Lives of Other Peoples

By Randall M. Packard
(Baltimore, MD: Johns Hopkins University Press, 2016)
(414 pages; $35.00 paper)

In his title, *A History of Global Health: Interventions into the Lives of Other Peoples*, Randall M. Packard introduces the thesis of his fine book: global health interventions have developed outside the countries involved, with little to no attempts to include local perspectives and community participation. These interventions have been remarkably constant over the 20th century, focusing on specific biomedical technologies and disease prevention measures that primarily ignore the social and economic determinants of health. With an assumption in the superiority of Western medicine, science, and technology, international health care leaders have discouraged longer-term interventions that build local health infrastructures. Packard does not deny that some improvement in health occurred, but interventions have had limited impact on overall health in many areas of the world.

Packard opens and closes the book with a discussion of Ebola as a case study of an epidemic in which interventions failed because of a lack of health care infrastructures. This absence stemmed from inattention to the social and economic causes of disease in the affected countries, which led to the epidemic in the first place. He then divides the book into seven parts organized chronologically. His writing is superb and his primary and secondary sources are numerous.

Part I begins with a historical analysis of colonial medicine and how it became entangled with the new field of international health. By describing William Gorgas and his work with yellow fever in the early 20th century in Cuba and Panama, Packard argues that US health authorities directly intervened in the lives of local populations. It was in these countries that medical science, disease eradication campaigns, and programs such as anti-mosquito efforts became the center of international health and continued to guide campaigns throughout the twentieth century. Colonial possessions "became training grounds for a generation of US public-health workers who would later take up positions in emerging international-health organizations" (p. 19). Indeed, workers in these early colonial campaigns became leaders in the programs of the Rockefeller Foundation International Health

Nursing History Review 27 (2019): 156–158. A Publication of the American Association for the History of Nursing. Copyright © 2019 Springer Publishing Company.
http://dx.doi.org/10.1891/1062-8061.27.156

Board. Health experts extended Rockefeller Foundation activities, honed in the campaign against hookworm in the southern part of the United States, to the American-occupied Philippines and to British colonial possessions in the Caribbean and South and East Asia. Treatment involved painful drugs and intrusive sanitation measures with no efforts to gain local cooperation. Campaigns aimed to obtain quick results and became an enduring goal of future health programs.

Parts II and III extend the analysis to the 1930s and 1940s. The 1930s were years of promise for an alternative approach to international health that addressed underlying social and economic determinants of health. Packard discusses the League of Nations Health Organization's broader vision to assist people out of poverty. As well, the Rockefeller Foundation's campaigns in China, Mexico, Java, and Ceylon were helpful as health care workers involved local leaders in a rural reconstruction program that focused on housing, agricultural development, and nutrition. In the aftermath of World War II, the United Nations Relief and Rehabilitation Administration focused on women and children and resurrected health services in war-torn Europe. That said, health leaders soon reverted back to the application of new biomedical technologies. New actors entered the scene, such as the World Health Organization (WHO), the World Bank, and the International Monetary Fund. By the 1950s, Africa, Asia, and Latin America became targets of their programs. In these countries, epidemics and famines led to a "perception of crisis" (p. 106), which continued the search for interventions that had quick biomedical solutions.

In Part IV, Packard describes the WHO's less-than-successful antimalarial campaign that focused on DDT spraying, which he contrasts with the organization's success in smallpox eradication. Through these case studies, he pushes his thesis that the campaigns involved the extension of public health technology and biomedicine by planners outside the countries involved.

Part V is particularly interesting for the author's analysis of population-control campaigns that took precedent in the 1960s, 1970s, and 1980s. He discusses the push for contraception, the WHO's development of family planning programs, and the opposition of the Catholic Church. This debate is one of Packard's few mentions of nurses, as he details the work of Puerto Rican nurses who "viewed family planning as a form of positive eugenics aimed at working-class women." They aimed to provide birth control in order to produce "the right sort of working-class family—small, nuclear, and legitimate" (p. 189).

The final parts of the book focus on the rise and fall of the primary health care model, AIDS, and the medicalizing of global health. In these sections,

Packard highlights two particularly interesting points. He argues that Bill and Melinda Gates have once again brought attention to the notion of disease eradication, a noble aim, but an approach that guided the Rockefeller Foundation in the 1920s and other international health organizations throughout the century. The belief is that new technologies and financial resources can make the dream of disease eradication possible. The second point is his discussion of the medicalization of global health. Citing a 1976 Millbank Fund report, schools of public health were becoming so dependent on research dollars that they no longer controlled their destinies. Today, rather than working on building and sustaining programs aimed at social determinants of health, public health students are being trained to expand their careers by doing biomedical research.

Currently, researchers are looking for a new vaccine against Ebola, but Packard's history of the circulation of biomedical ideas and people across the globe has a warning: Finding vaccines and providing medicines do save lives, but they "delay efforts to build health systems and alleviate the structural causes of disease" (p. 341). This limited vision should be a lesson for us all.

I highly recommend the book for health professionals, global health workers, policy leaders, and academic departments in global health, history, sociology, and public health.

Barbra Mann Wall, PhD, RN, FAAN
University of Virginia
225 Jeanette Lancaster Way
Charlottesville, VA 22903

Madhouse: Psychiatry and Politics in Cuban History

By Jennifer L. Lambe
(Chapel Hill, NC: The University of North Carolina Press, 2017)
(344 pages; $90.00 cloth, $32.95 paper, $19.99 e-book)

The *Hospital Psiquiátrico de La Habana*, known to generations of Cubans simply as *Mazorra*, after the eponymous slave trader upon whose land the institution was built in the 19th century, has been a fixture in the Cuban psyche since its founding. Publicly and privately, Cubans have long characterized Mazorra as everything from a symbol of Cuban progress to a Dantesque inferno. Lost in this formulation has been the complex history of the institution and of the burgeoning mental health fields that sprouted up alongside it on the island. Jennifer Lambe's sweeping and erudite monograph not only provides a fascinating account of Mazorra's history but also reframes the institution, and indeed Cuban psychiatric and psychological research and practice, as prime sites of contestation over key themes in Cuba's history including imperialism, modernity, race, gender, and revolution.

In the waning years of the empire, Spanish officials viewed Mazorra as little more than a dumping ground for Cuba's castoffs: the mentally ill, criminals, the aged, and former slaves. When US forces took formal possession of Cuba in 1899, the asylum was, like much of the island, shattered by hunger and staggering neglect. Lambe points out that during this period Mazorra quickly became something more than just an asylum. It offered American officials—especially those deeply influenced by Progressivism—an opportunity to demonstrate a brand of imperialism imbued with notions of "compassionate governance" (p. 21). For Cubans, just as significantly, it became "a vital nationalist project, a rejection of the horrors of the past" (p. 20). Under the leadership of the Dr. Lucas Álvarez Cerice, Mazorra's historic position as a "carceral asylum" would change (p. 33). Álvarez Cerice reformed patient care, improved housing, and created a cadre of nurses specially trained in mental health. Mazorra became not just a model of public medical care on the island but also an emblem of the fledgling Cuban republic's march toward modernity.

Despite these successes, however, Mazorra perpetually fell victim to the corruption that seemingly infused every part of Cuban political life in the early decades of the republic. Lambe shows how the asylum became a source of sinecures (Cuba's notorious *botella* system), how administrators exploited its patients for their labor, and, disturbingly, how inmates' bodies, particularly those of black women, were used by Cuban researchers to conduct experiments in fields such as gynecology. The Cuban press feasted on accounts of abuse at the institution and successive generations of opportunistic Cuban political leaders would point to it as a primary target for "revolutionary ablution" (p. 113).

Yet, *Madhouse* is more than a history of Mazorra. Lambe employs the asylum as a springboard from which to examine the fraught history of psychiatry and psychology in Cuban culture and politics. The identification and treatment of mental illness became important in Cuba in the 1940s and 1950s as the government expanded services for the poor and wealthier Cubans began to fill the offices of private *consultas* in Havana, storming "their doctors offices in search of Oedipal conflicts" (p. 123). The effort to bring psychiatric order to the nation, however, often involved taking aim at various "deviant" sexual practices including homosexuality. Building on a rich archive of patient studies published in Cuba's robust medical press, Lambe shows how psychiatry was deployed to control women's bodies and behavior and, in a culture powerfully shaped by patriarchy and heternormativity, also pathologized homosexuals.

The final chapters of *Madhouse* are finely executed and place psychiatry and shifting notions of mental illness, and indeed conceptions of sanity, at the center of the tumultuous Cuban Revolution. Fidel Castro, like generations of earlier Cuban revolutionaries, promised to redeem Mazorra and its patients. "The Hospital Psiquiátrico," Lambe writes, "represented nothing less than a laboratory for revolutionary process, a crucible of the human experiment that the Revolution had inaugurated" (p. 141). But it wasn't just Mazorra, rechristened by the Revolution as the *Hospital Psiquiátrico de la Habana*, that underwent a transformation. Psychiatric practice too was realigned, often uneasily, with revolutionary processes and goals. This realignment put Cuban mental health professionals in an awkward and sometimes dangerous place and revealed that very often "state prerogatives trumped psychiatric knowledge" (p. 195).

Lambe has produced an impressive volume that offers a number of important lines for further investigation including the causes of Mazorra's late imperial decline. This well-written and impressively researched book will become a foundational text in the history of Cuban medicine and disease.

Madhouse will be of interest to historians of Latin America and the Caribbean and historians of medicine and disease and is accessible to upper-level undergraduates and graduate students.

JOHN A. GUTIÉRREZ
Assistant Professor
Department of Latin American and Latina/o Studies
John Jay College of Criminal Justice/CUNY
524 West 59th Street, 8th Floor
New York, NY 10019

Toxic Exposures: Mustard Gas and the Health
Consequences of World War II in the United States
By Susan L. Smith
(New Brunswick, NJ: Rutgers University Press, 2017)
(200 pages; $29.95 cloth/e-book)

In *Toxic Exposures*, Susan L. Smith examines the history and legacies of mustard gas experiments conducted in the name of wartime preparation and weapons development during and after the World War II. It is a medical history of mustard gas according to Smith, one that reveals the health consequences of wartime medical research. While Great Britain, Australia, and Canada, U.S. allies during World War II, figure as part of the story, this is predominately a transnational history of the United States' relationship to mustard gas. Smith ultimately argues that "mustard gas was, and still is, a defining feature of the war's legacy for soldiers' health, racialized science, ocean environments, and cancer treatments in the United States," … a history that demonstrates how advances in medical knowledge and protections to national security came at the cost of human rights (p. 3).

Smith has a broad agenda for such a slim volume at 200 pages. The book is organized in two parts thematically and chronologically with the addition of both an introduction and conclusion. In Part I, Smith "investigates the preparation for chemical warfare through mustard gas experiments on servicemen, including race-based toxicity studies" (p. 10). Over the course of two chapters, Smith focused on how medical research was ostensibly used for military benefits. Mustard gas experiments were, "part of the militarization of medicine and the medicalization of war" (p. 21). This relationship between the military and medicine is important for two reasons. First, it reveals how soldiers on the home front, according to Smith, became as important to the war effort, although certainly less known, as those fighting overseas. In this way, Smith focus' on home front soldiering fits within a larger body of scholarship on work within the context of wartime.

Second, Smith's focus on the relationship between the military and medicine also reveals how chemical warfare research in support of the war effort "contributed to racism in the United States" (p. 45). Chapter 2 exposes how scientists began conducting race studies as part of their mustard gas experiments. Readers will expect to find information about studies conducted on African American soldiers and it is here in abundance. However,

Nursing History Review 27 (2019): 162–164. A Publication of the American Association for the History of Nursing. Copyright © 2019 Springer Publishing Company.
http://dx.doi.org/10.1891/1062-8061.27.162

Smith expands this conversation to show how scientists also used Japanese Americans, Puerto Ricans, and Panamanians in their attempted to understand how different bodies reacted to mustard gas and how these differences might be exploited in the use of chemical weapons against allied enemies. This chapter will be especially attractive to those scholars interested in examining another way that race shaped medical knowledge during World War II.

In Part II, "Toxic Legacies of War," Smith considers the "toxic health legacies of mustard gas in relation to ocean pollution and cancer treatments." It is in this section of the text that Smith's work really shines. Both chapters highlight how toxicity was not just destructive but also served as a constructive foundation for environmental protection and medical advances. Chapter 3, "Mustard Gas in the Sea Around Us," explores the history of dumping mustard gas around the globe and off the coasts of North America. Here, Smith reveals how the legacy of mustard gas is connected to, and part of, larger conversations about the environmental impact of waging war. Using the work of environmental activists such as Rachel Carson and Jacques Cousteau Smith shows that it was not just servicemen but civilians and the environment that also continue to deal with the hazards of mustard gas and other weapons of war. In Chapter 4, "A Wartime Story," Smith illuminates how war supported and even encouraged scientists to expand medical knowledge. In other words, mustard gas experiments made it possible for doctors to apply the knowledge from the experiments to the "problem of cancer" using chemical treatments (p. 114).

Smith concludes the narrative with a conversation on the ongoing challenges faced by veterans attempting to gain both recognition for their work as soldiers and support for their long-term health problems from their toxic exposure to mustard gas. It is here and in the previous two chapters that Smith narrative is the strongest, exposing the expansive legacies of chemical research and use. If the book falls short in any way it is in the repetition of the author's arguments in the first two chapters of the narrative; however, the brevity of the work would appeal to a broad range of scholars and to professors looking to introduce their student to topics such as chemical warfare and wartime research, civil–military relations, race, environmentalism, and health activism.

CHARISSA THREAT, PhD
Assistant Professor of History
Spelman College
350 Spelman Lane, SW Box 823
Atlanta, GA 30314-4399

Ebola: How a People's Science Helped End an Epidemic

By Paul Richards
(London, UK: ZED Books, 2016)
(180 pages; $24.95 paperback)

From his own perspective as an anthropologist in Sierra Leone, author Paul Richards describes and analyzes the local and international response to the horrific outbreak of the Ebola virus that swept through West Africa in 2013 and 2014. In this book, he argues that the "emergent disease" that began at the forest edge in Guinea was "less a disease of poverty than a disease of ignorance" (p. 7) and that shared perspectives, from the world health community and that of the "common folk" on the ground, was key to its eradication. "What mattered," according to Richards, "was the extent to which communities at risk of Ebola were capable of recognizing the risks posed by their existing embodied practices and to elaborate safer techniques" (p. 28).

While Richard's analysis has some truth, particularly (1) the need for experts to understand the local cultural practices and (2) the fact that people responding to emergent diseases should maintain open channels of communication between communities and themselves, the book has several limitations. Chief among these is the author's perspective as an anthropologist rather than a physician, public health expert, or historian. The fact that Richards does not use accurate descriptors (this was a *pandemic,* not an epidemic for example, and *can* be treated—in first-world countries with high tech, scientific interventions) is not only distracting to the reader who is aware of the science behind Ebola, but also undermines the credibility of the book's thesis. Moreover, Richard's awkward attempt to overlay theoretical frameworks from anthropology (e.g. Durkheim, Mauss, Geertz, the Hewletts), and his use of academic jargon in sentences like: "Techniques of the body need to be understood as essential human resources in the co-production of material and social life" (p. 67)—when referring to nursing and burial practices—interfere with the readability of the book. There is no coherent narrative describing the "who, what, where, and when" of the pandemic; nor does the author take into account aspects of race, class, and gender, as one would expect from any historian discussing this public health emergency. Clearly, the fact that Ebola occurred in a third-world country with inadequate medical and transportation infrastructure, poverty, and a lack of scientific knowledge among the local people had a major impact on the progression of the disease. It also affected

Nursing History Review 27 (2019): 165–166. A Publication of the American Association for the History of Nursing. Copyright © 2019 Springer Publishing Company.
http://dx.doi.org/10.1891/1062-8061.27.165

the international response. The same could be said for the invisibility of local health care responders: class and race mattered. As Barbra Mann Wall and I note in our book *Nurses and Disasters*: As of August 2014, 15 *African* nurses had died—risking their lives to work on the front lines of the battle against Ebola. Yet they remain anonymous, most likely because of their race and their homeland. It was only when two white American nurses contracted Ebola in Dallas, Texas, that the risk to nurses was taken seriously at an international level.[1]

In addition to factual inaccuracies, Richard's writing style leaves much to be desired. His frequent references to what he will discuss in future chapters, for example, is distracting and evidence of a hurried project. The same could be said for the contradictions within the text: at one point he says the local community sought instruction in safe burial techniques, only to say at another point that the government's law making washing a corpse a "criminal offense punishable by two years in jail" (p. 52) may have done more harm than good. In other sections, he changes his purpose/argument. The book should have been a page-turner and it is not. A good editor could have strengthened this work significantly.

All that having been said, the book does capture some of the complexities of the world health response to an emergent disease in a developing nation, and highlights the importance of understanding local culture and its health and burial processes in responding to such an emergency. As for the audience likely to benefit from the book, Richards notes that it targets "citizens of the world who have an interest in the health of their global neighbors" (p. 9).

Note

1. For additional perspective on this, see: Arlene Keeling and Barbra Mann Wall, (eds.) Preface to *Nurses and Disasters: Global, Historical Case Studies* (New York: Springer Publishing, 2015): xi–xii. See also: Barbra Mann Wall, Editorial, "Supporting the Ebola Nurses," in *Health, Emergency, and Disaster Nursing*, 2, (2015): 1–2.

ARLENE W. KEELING, PHD, RN, FAAN
Professor Emerita
The University of Virginia School of Nursing
225 Jeanette Lancaster Way
Charlottesville, VA 22903

Hurt: The Inspiring, Untold Story of Trauma Care

By Catherine Musemeche
(Lebanon, NH: ForeEdge, University Press of New England, 2016)
(268 pages; $27.95 cloth, $22.99 e-book)

In the introduction to the book, author Catherine Musemeche promises to tell "the story of how trauma care evolved into the effective system that it is today and the dedicated men and women who helped build it" (p. 1). Traumatic injuries and events touch lives around the world daily, and in the United States injuries are the leading cause of disability for individuals under 65 years old and the leading cause of death for children and adolescents. Accidents, wars, natural disasters, and violence have always been (and will continue to be) relevant, and Musemeche aims to take the reader on a journey through the groundbreaking discoveries that have driven the science of trauma care forward. In an interview about her book, Musemeche states "I see my job as a writer to take a complicated topic like operating on babies or trauma care and distill it down to concepts any reader can understand and also to illustrate the drama and high stakes involved in medical practice."[1] With this context in mind, this book has accomplished the goals of the author; however, this book fails to meet the expectations of its stated purpose to explain the full history of the evolution of the trauma system from its beginnings to its current state.

The evidence used to support her work mostly comes from published articles, biographies, websites, and newspaper articles, and is lacking in archival sources. She pulls from her own experience as a pediatric surgeon, as well as the experience of famous and little-known victims of trauma to dramatize the story. The book lacks focus and includes rather varied topics, such as pre-hospital cardiac care, wilderness medicine, and a discussion of gun control laws. While interesting, these topics are tangentially related to the history of trauma and do not support the purpose of her book, nor illustrate the evolution of trauma care. In explaining an "evolving trauma system," Musemeche fails to create a tangible historical thread and does not explain how the facts and developments mentioned in separate chapters connect to the larger story of the development of trauma. As a nurse, I was disappointed that nurses were largely absent from Musemeche's history of trauma care, with the exception of Elizabeth Scanlon, who assisted Dr. Cowley in his research on shock. Musemeche's illustration of trauma care is one-dimensional, and largely misses the interdisciplinary nature of trauma across the continuum of care, in which

Nursing History Review 27 (2019): 167–169. A Publication of the American Association for the History of Nursing. Copyright © 2019 Springer Publishing Company.
http://dx.doi.org/10.1891/1062-8061.27.167

physicians, nurses, and a variety of allied health professionals from multiple specialties are absolutely critical.

Hurt is organized in three sections: pre-hospital care, treatment of traumatic injuries, and rehabilitation. Each chapter is organized around a theme related to trauma, such as the impact of blood banking, treating traumatic brain injury, or the development of the science of injury prevention. These chapters all contain compelling personal stories of patients and physicians who have benefitted from these advancements in trauma, surrounded by an often superficial appraisal of the historical development of these advances. *Hurt* is not a scholarly history of trauma care. Musemeche's biographical approach focuses on hand-picked leaders and pioneers in the field, praising their accomplishments rather than critically examining the socio-political forces that contributed to the establishment of a trauma system in the United States.

Noticeably missing is a discussion on the impact of race, gender, or social class on trauma treatment. The author celebrates Phil Hallen as a Yale-educated hospital administrated who founded an ambulance service to "put young men of color to work" in the "impoverished African American inner-city neighborhood known as the Hill District," (p. 64) creating the Freedom House Ambulance Service. Musemeche misses an opportunity to discuss the accomplishments of these men as pioneers in prehospital care, and instead focuses on Hallen and the medical director, Dr. Peter Safar. Musemeche recognizes the research of Dr. R. Adams Cowley, the founder of the modern-day trauma system, and the work he completed in his "death lab" at the University of Maryland at Baltimore. She neglects to mention the disparaging human cost of this research. Most of those living in the area surrounding this urban, academic medical center in the 1960s (and today) were poor African Americans, and would have been the most likely participants in his research.

Although entertaining, this book is more appropriate for the casual reader who is interested in trauma, rather than a medical professional or scholar engaged in this type of work. If read in isolation, each chapter is an engaging celebration of select pioneers who have furthered each specific concept of trauma care. The reader can learn about Sue Baker, the epidemiologist responsible for groundbreaking research in the realm of injury prevention, or Dr. Spurgeon Neel, a pioneer in medical evacuation by helicopter. Readers can be inspired by the surgical excellence of military and civilian physicians saving their patient's life when all hope seemed lost, and finish the book with a hodgepodge of interesting facts about amputations or modern advances in spinal cord repair. If you are interested in a light, easy to read, entertaining, and engaging collection of trauma stories, this is the book for you. However, if you were looking for a critical, comprehensive, or scholarly approach to the history of trauma, I would recommend reading a different book.

Note

1. *The Librarian Talks*, "Interview: Catherine Musemeche, MD on *HURT: The Inspiring, Untold Story of Trauma Care*," *The Librarian Talks*, October 3, 2016, accessed February 26, 2018, https://thelibrariantalks.wordpress.com/2016/10/03/interview-catherine-musemeche-md-on-hurt-the-inspiring-untold-story-of-trauma-care/.

GWYNETH MILBRATH, PhD, RN, MPH
Clinical Assistant Professor
University of Illinois Chicago College of Nursing
845 S. Damen Ave, MC 802
Chicago, IL 60612-7350

History of Professional Nursing in the United States: Toward a Culture of Health

By Arlene W. Keeling, Michelle C. Hehman, and John C. Kirchgessner
(New York, NY: Springer Publishing Company, 2018)
(391 pages; $85.00 paperback)

For many, history of nursing publications have been a compendium of the "usual suspects" of familiar and notable figures in nursing. This is not to detract from the critically important role that these trailblazing and far-seeing individuals have imprinted on the development of modern nursing. Critical analysis, however, demands that the history of nursing is not series of singular discrete persons who have placed their stamp on this profession, but to also address nursing from varying perspectives. The *History of Professional Nursing in the United States: Toward a Culture of Health* by Arlene W. Keeling, Michelle C. Hehman, and John C. Kirchgessner utilizes the concept of both U.S. nursing as well as health promotion as guides in this book. And they have succeeded brilliantly in portraying nursing not as just a healing profession, but one that seeks to promote health through varying components of social determinants of health in combination with contemporary knowledge of technology that is shaping the continually evolving nature of professional nursing. The authors acknowledge Nightingale in the clever "what it is" and "what it is not" by asserting that this book does not seek to be a comprehensive history of nursing and health care because it focuses on efforts in the United States. It also seeks to redress nursing history's more familiar perspective of white middle-class women to recognize the work of others representing varied ethnicities, classes, and gender who provided leadership in nursing, be it through education or clinical practice. The 15 chapters span the Colonial era to the challenges of promoting and sustaining a culture of health in the 21st century. Each chapter expands on a theme, from roots (Chapter 2), to early 20th-century innovation (Chapter 6), seminal historic events (Chapters 8–11), as well as resulting changes that occurred from these events (Chapters 12–13). Recent crisis events are addressed through this lens (Chapter 14) and how this then challenges nursing as it moves forward (Chapter 15). The *History of Professional Nursing in the United States: Toward a Culture of Health* is not presenting new and original scholarship, but draws upon previously published content using health promotion as the framework. Keeling, Hehman, and Kirchgessner provide a fresh perspective to nursing history through their analysis of health determinants, the many who have played a role to improve

Nursing History Review 27 (2019): 170–171. A Publication of the American Association for the History of Nursing. Copyright © 2019 Springer Publishing Company.
http://dx.doi.org/10.1891/1062-8061.27.170

health, and the long-lasting results of their efforts. This book represents the "it takes a village" approach to nursing history in the United States. It is a fascinating overview of how this profession has evolved in the United States, but more importantly, presents it through an innovative and exciting perspective to view nursing in a vibrant historical and influential context. It is a must-read for those who respect historical analysis in many guises, but also is one that needs to be included in any professional nursing course, be it undergraduate or graduate level, to highlight and reveal the myriad roles nurses had and continue to have.

TERESA M. O'NEILL, PhD
Professor Emerita
University of Holy Cross
New Orleans, LA

Fast Facts About the Nursing Profession: Historical Perspectives in a Nutshell

By Deborah Dolan Hunt
(New York, NY: Springer Publishing Company, 2017)
(154 pages; $35.00 paperback)

Recognizing the need for history content in nursing curricula and a need for an up-to-date nursing history text addressing contemporary professional issues, Deborah Dolan Hunt has compiled key facts about the nursing profession's history—facts that are readily available in one volume and that provide a comprehensive, albeit brief historical overview. Using extensive primary and secondary resources Dolan Hunt discusses how nursing care has been provided over millennia from the ancient Egyptian, Greek, and Roman civilizations to the 21st century. The book's chapters are organized following a social history model and include the contextual history of each chapter's era, illustrating how policy, science, medicine, and culture influenced, and are intertwined with, nursing's history. Although at times, facts are stated without the necessary contextual background thus leading the reader to question why or how the facts are relevant.

Throughout the book, the profession's leaders and their contributions to health care are also highlighted. There is a heavy emphasis on the history of nursing in the United States, however Dolan Hunt has expanded the breadth of the profession's history to include historical facts on nursing in Europe, Asia, and Africa. Enduring issues that have challenged the profession's leaders throughout its history are also addressed, including the various levels of entry into practice and the academic degrees associated with the profession. One issue that has persisted, continues to be, and is not addressed to any extent is the lack of diversity within the profession. While various cultures are addressed there is little mention of the contributions various minorities have made to the profession. Despite its brevity, the book does meet the author's goal and provides readily available facts about the nursing profession in a chronological and topical format—which in itself can be challenging, especially when considering the timeframe it covers. The book does reveal the profession's rich history and can be especially useful to non-nurses and those who are just entering the nursing profession. As a stand-alone text it may not be adequate in a nursing education environment, however, it is a valuable text

Nursing History Review 27 (2019): 172–173. A Publication of the American Association for the History of Nursing. Copyright © 2019 Springer Publishing Company.
http://dx.doi.org/10.1891/1062-8061.27.172

that can be used in combination with in-depth readings and lectures on the profession's history.

JOHN C. KIRCHGESSNER, PhD, RN
Associate Professor of Nursing
Wegmans School of Nursing
3690 East Avenue
Rochester, NY 14618

NEW DISSERTATIONS

Compiled for the Nursing History Review by Cynthia Connolly, PhD, RN, FAAN, Associate Editor of the *Nursing History Review* and Associate Professor, University of Pennsylvania School of Nursing, Philadelphia, PA. These dissertations can be obtained through Proquest Dissertations.

William R. Feeney, "Manifestations of the Maimed: The Perception of Wounded Soldiers in the Civil War North," 2015, PhD dissertation, West Virginia University. (Publication Number: 3741911).

Amanda L. Mahoney, "Careful and Complete Observation of the Patient: Nurses and the Sociotechnical System of Medical Research, 1930-1962," 2016, PhD dissertation, University of Pennsylvania. (Publication Number: 10120658).

Nursing History Review 27 (2019): 174. A Publication of the American Association for the History of Nursing. Copyright © 2019 Springer Publishing Company.
http://dx.doi.org/10.1891/1062-8061.27.174